Creative Coloring Mandalas for Adult Stress Less Coloring

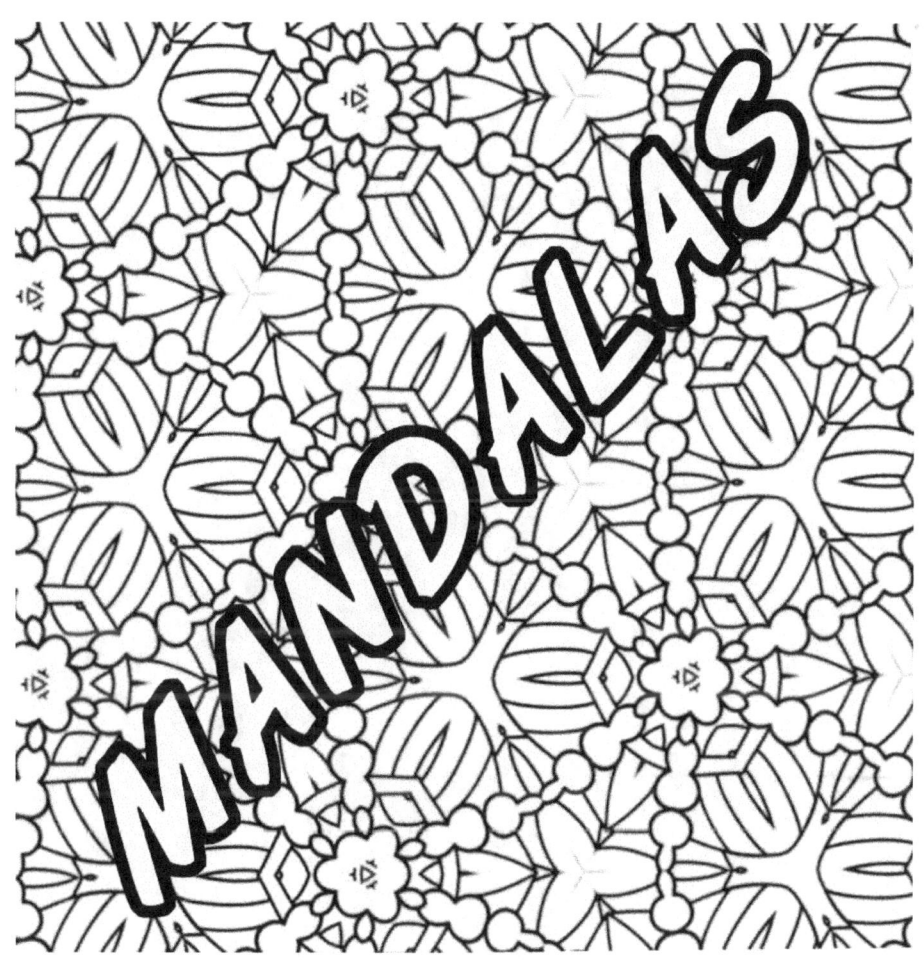

Jasmine Andrews

Creative Coloring Mandalas for Adult Stress Less Coloring

ISBN-13: 978-1543161830
ISBN-10: 1543161839

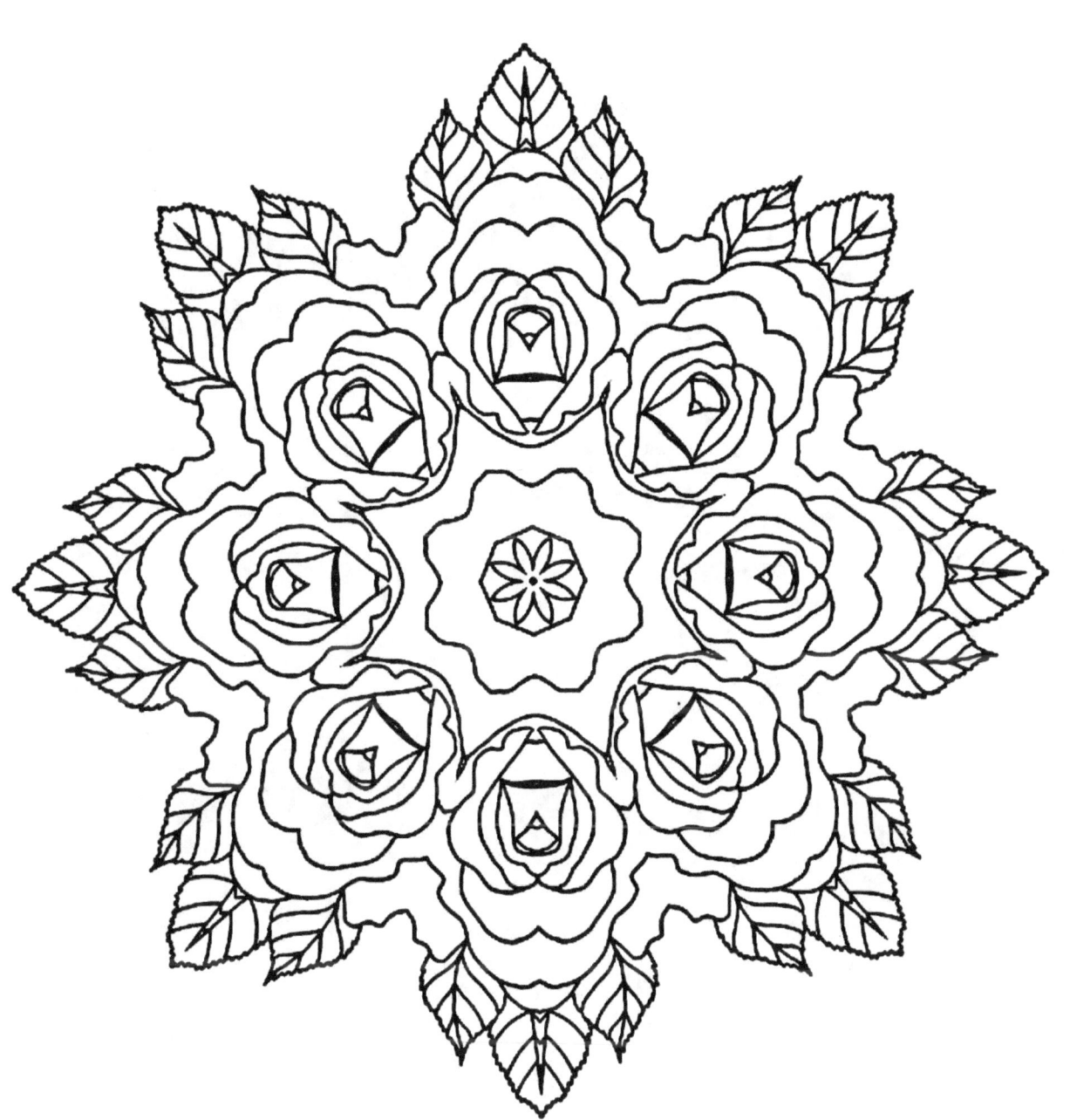

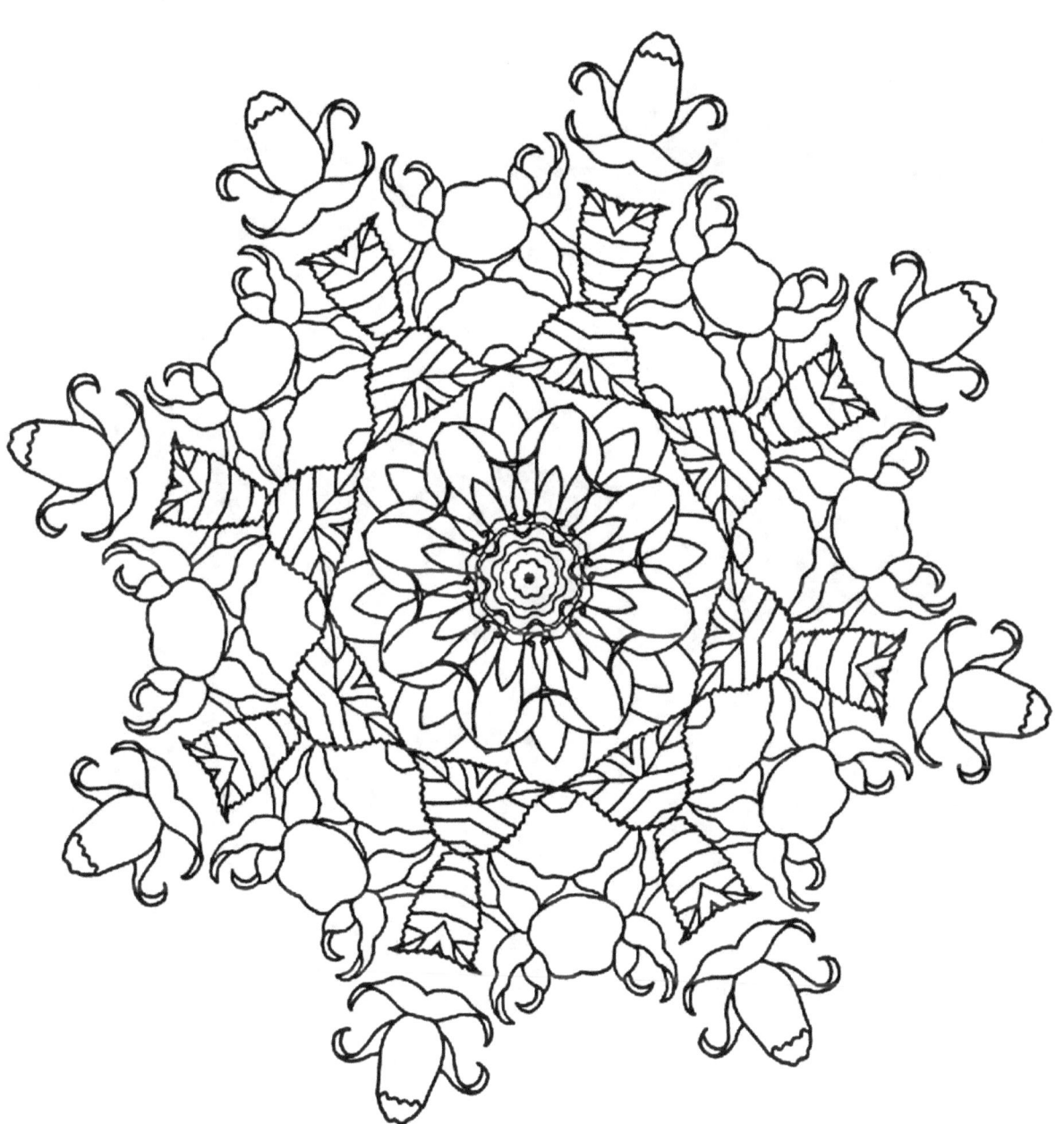

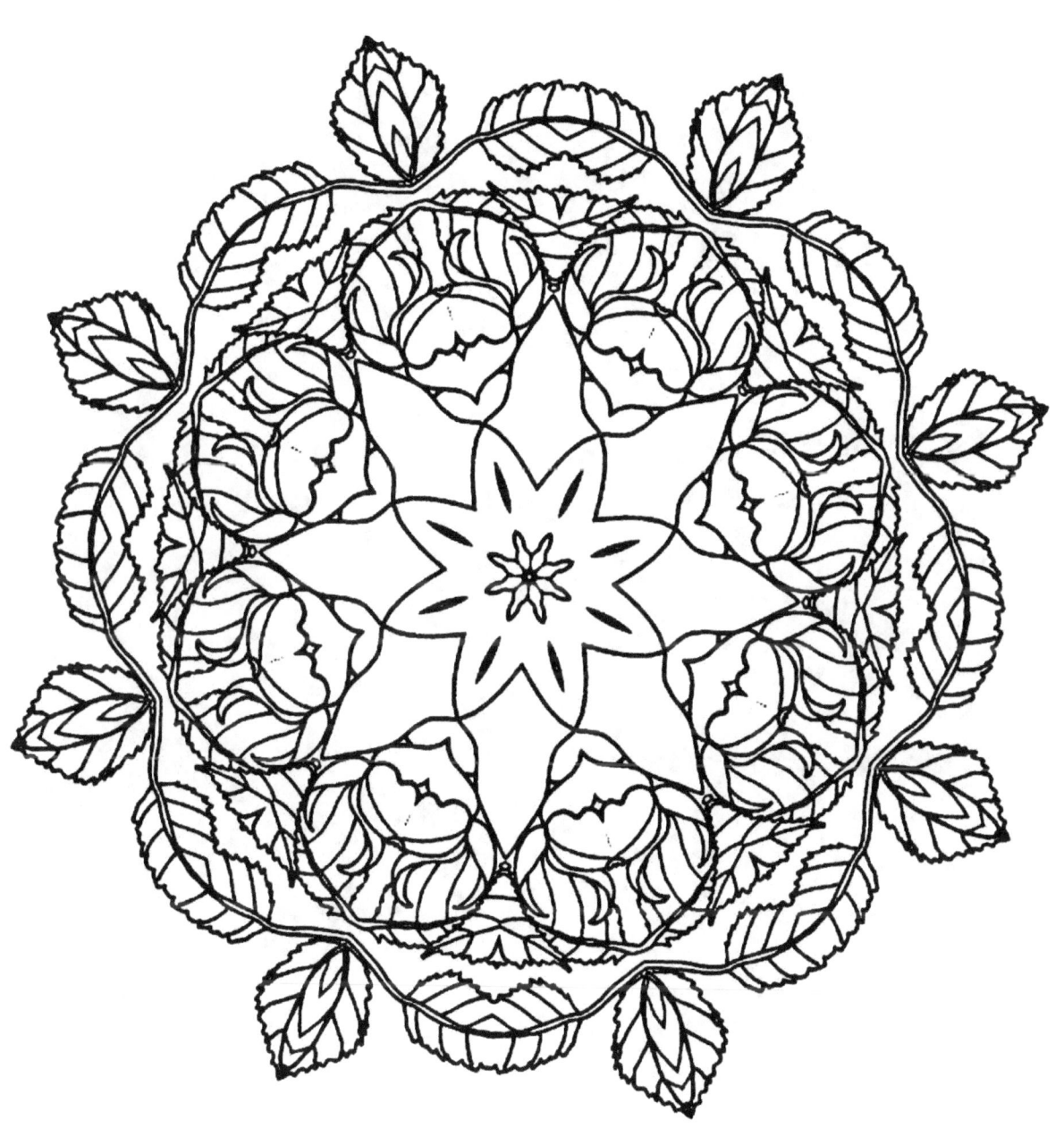

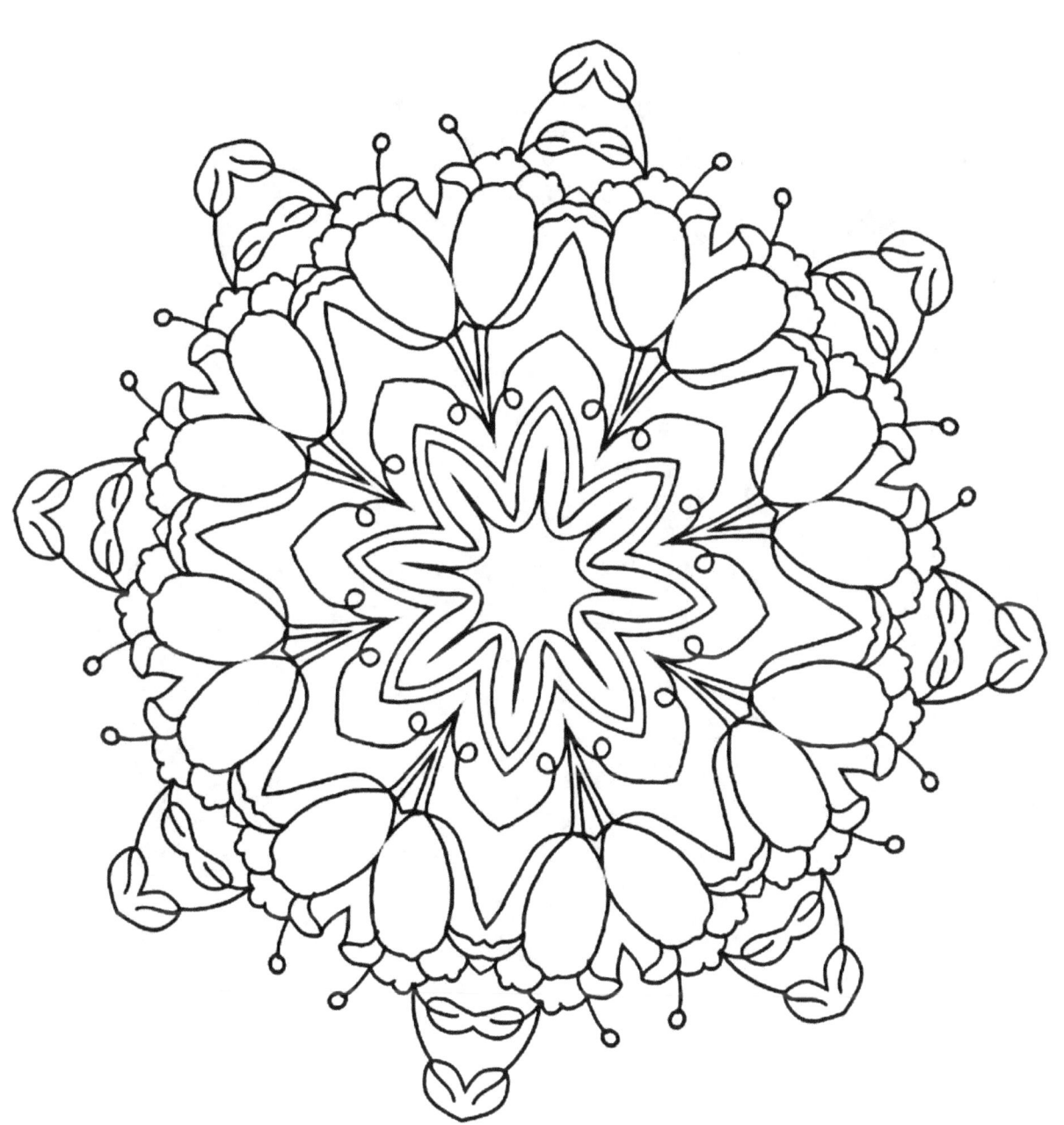

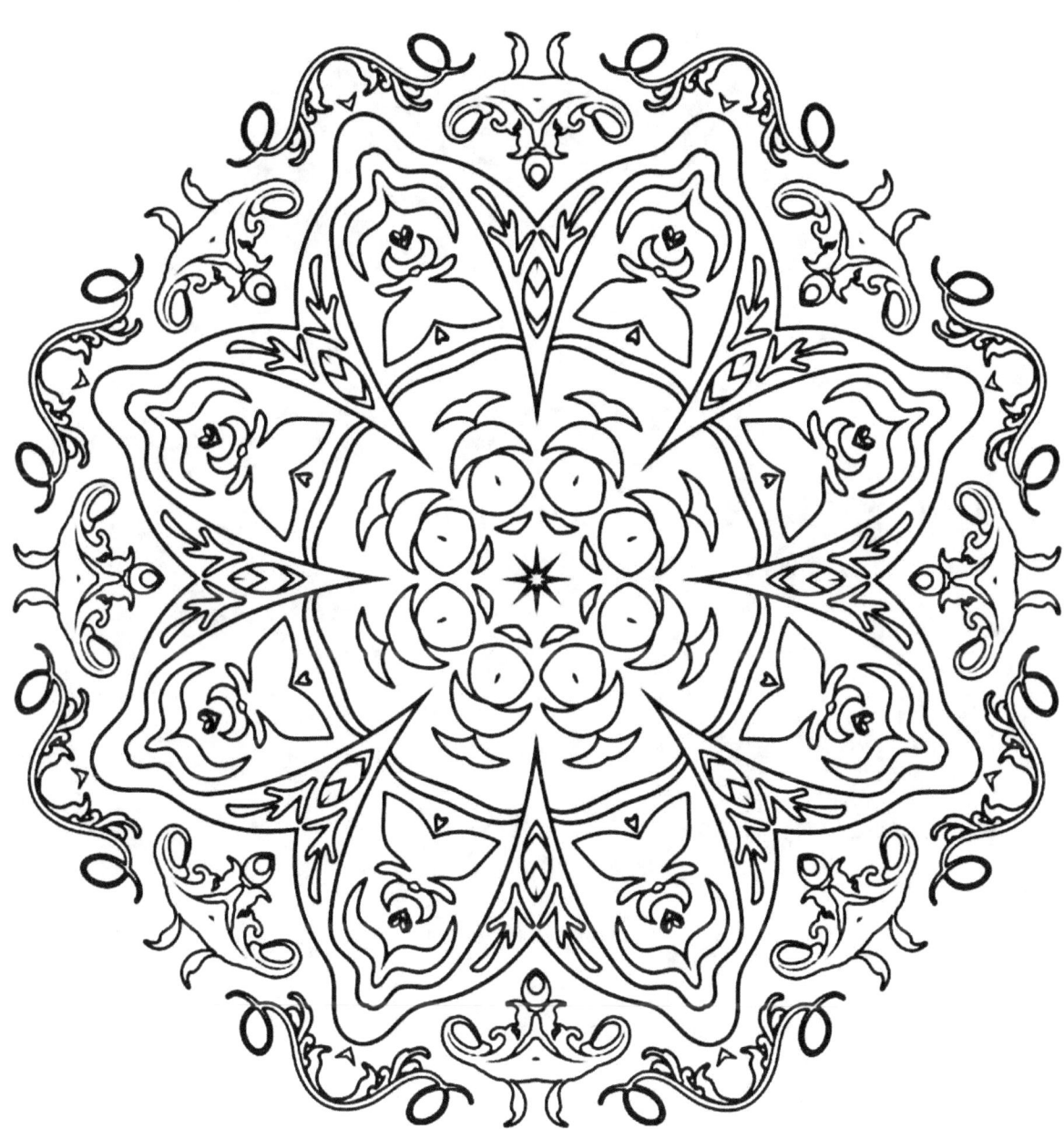

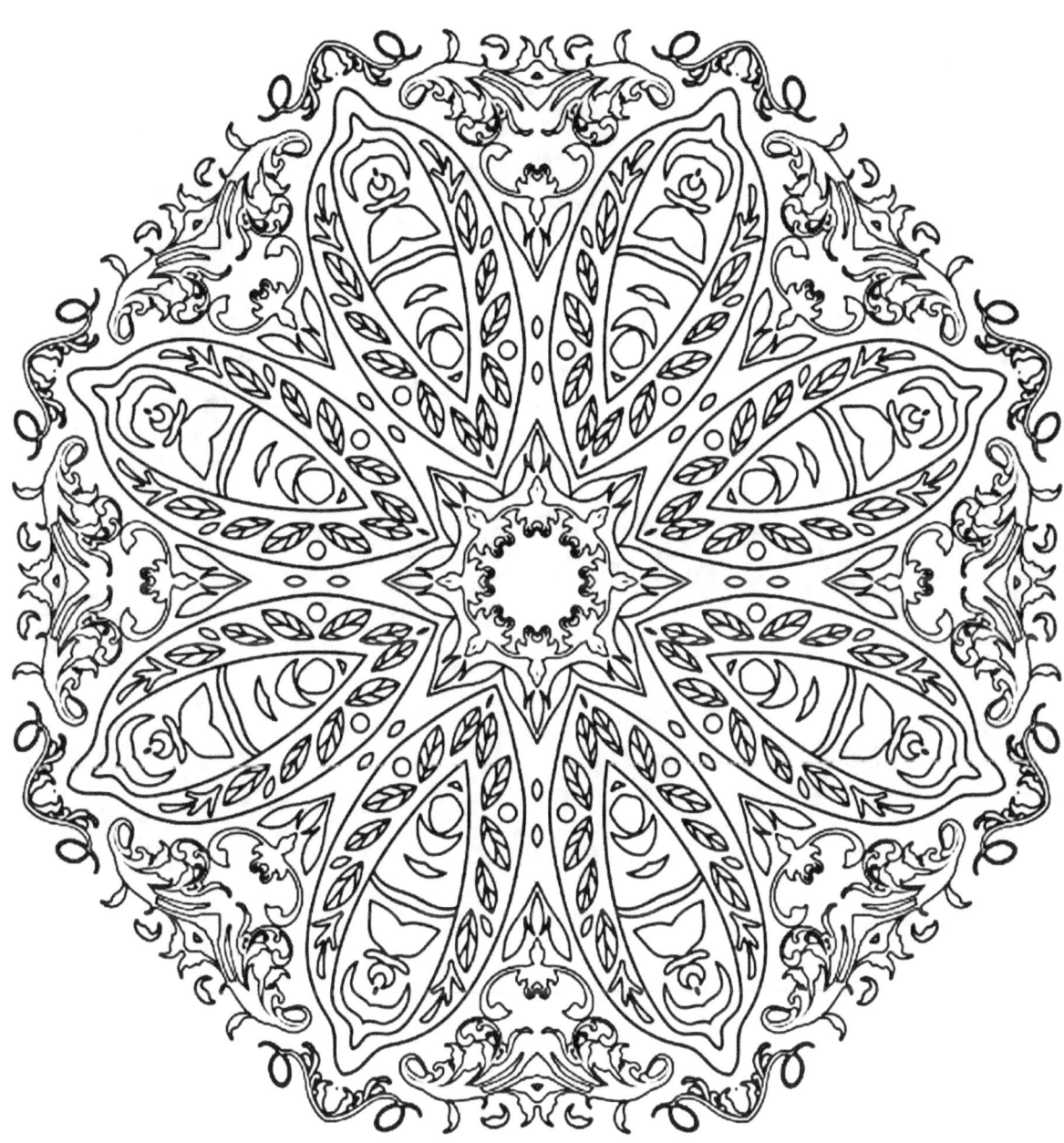

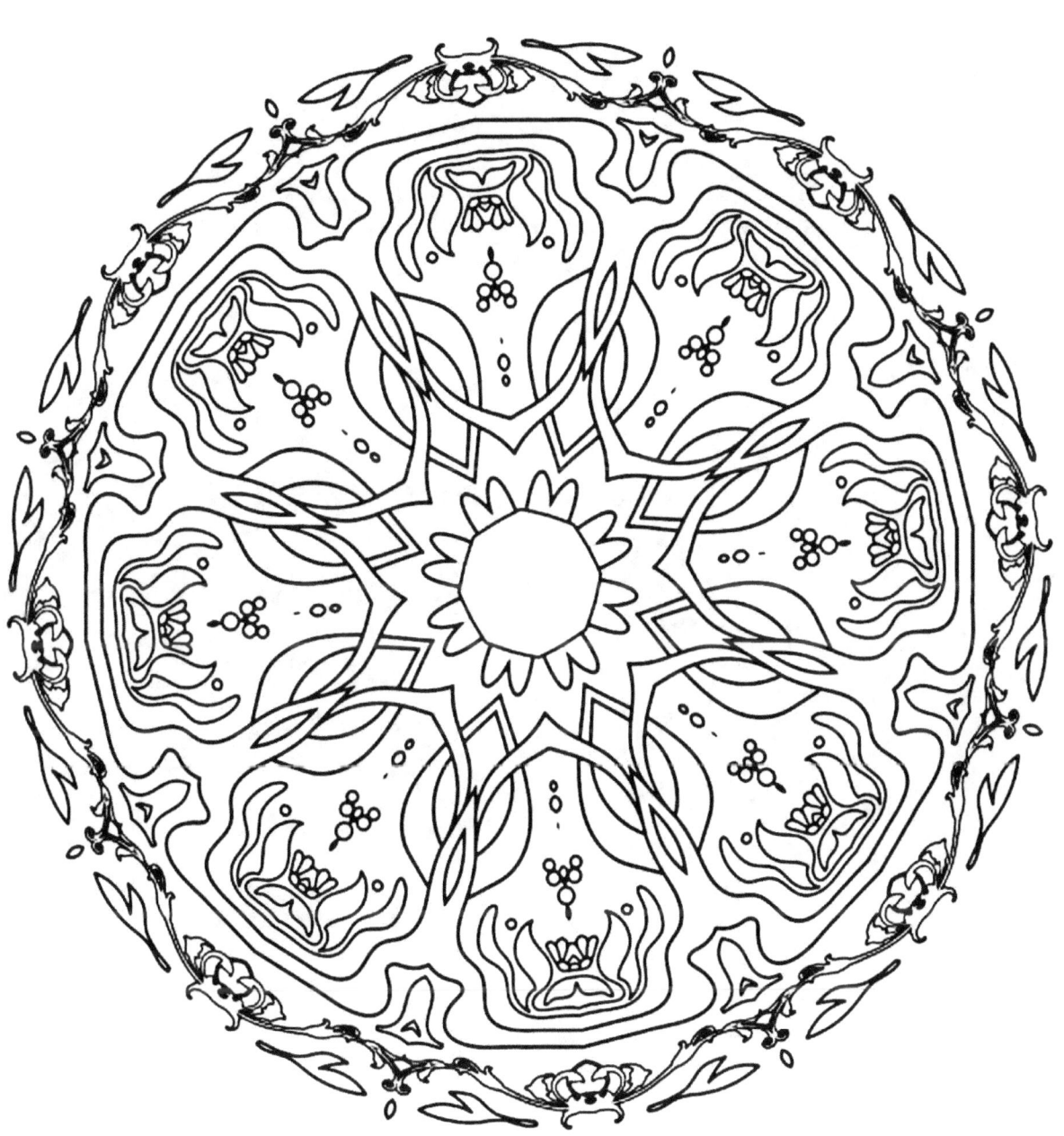

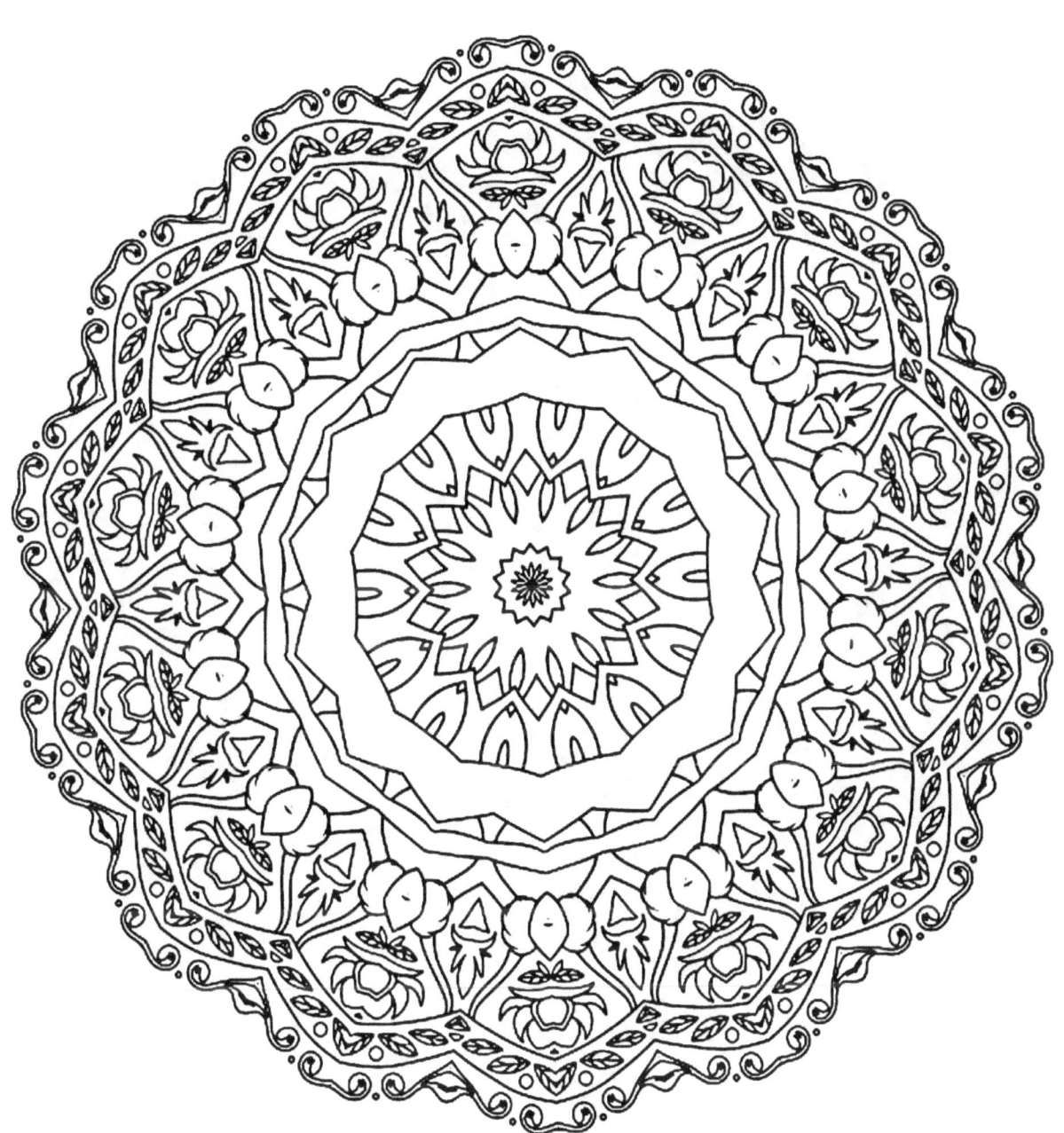

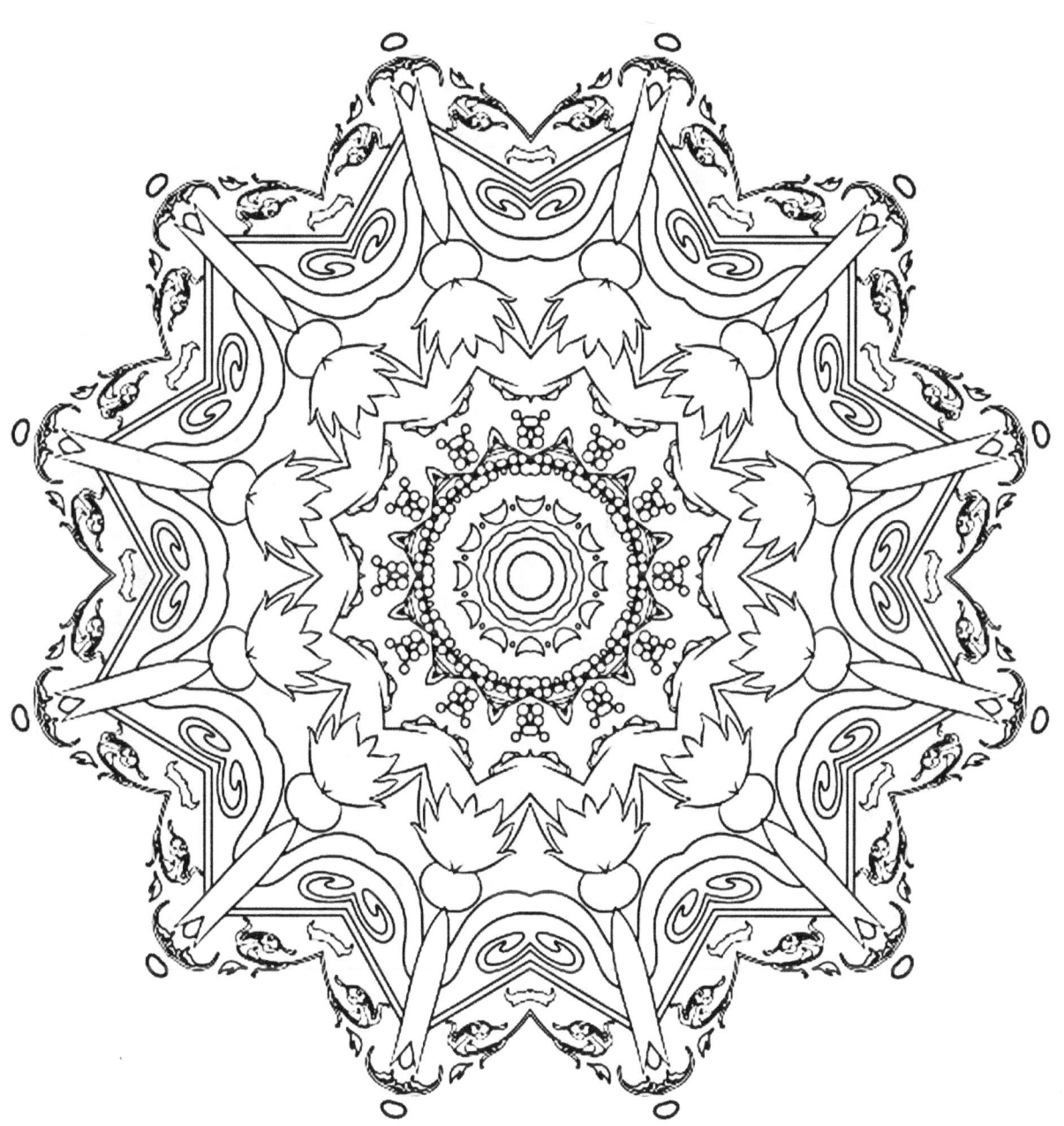

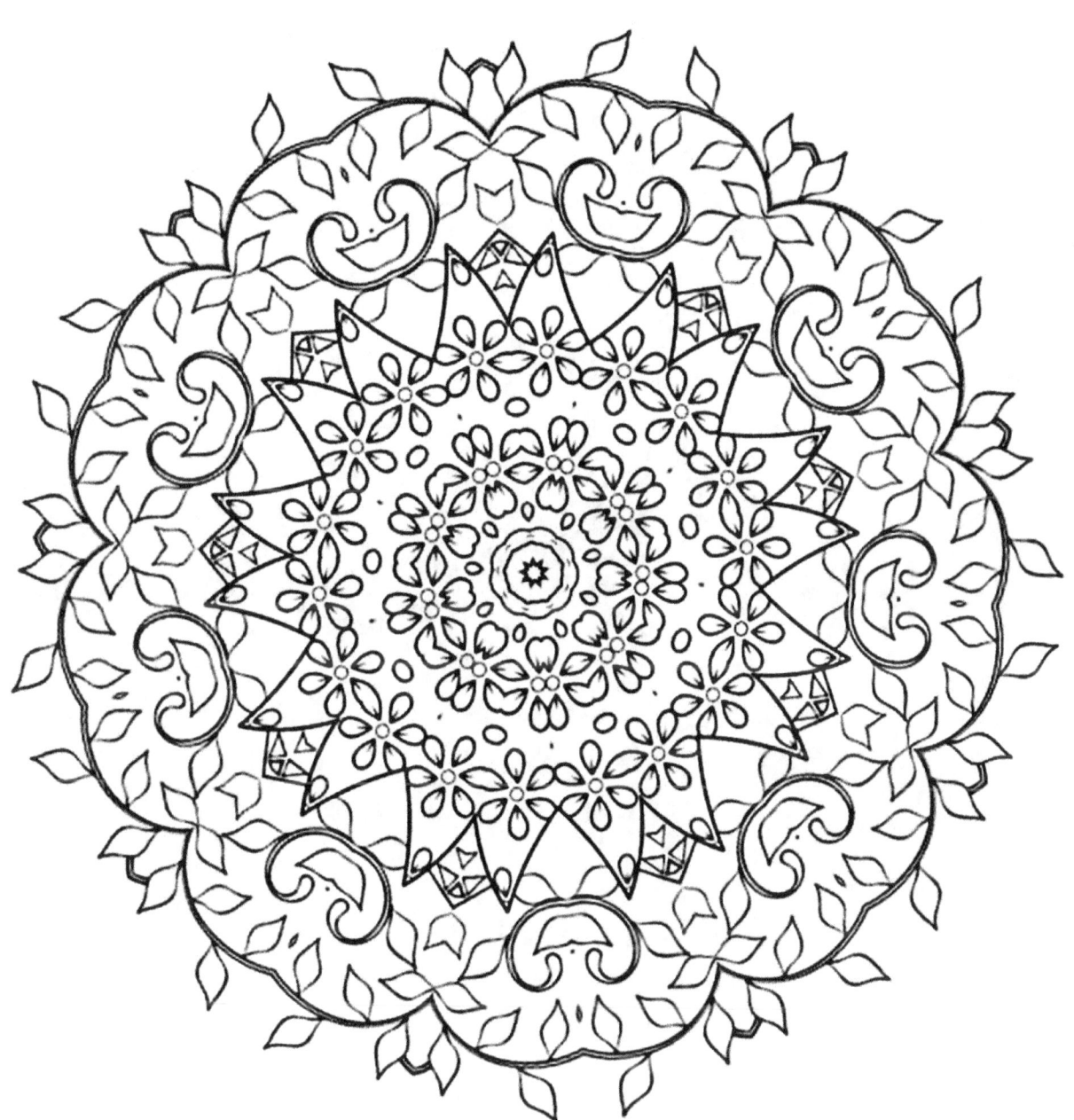

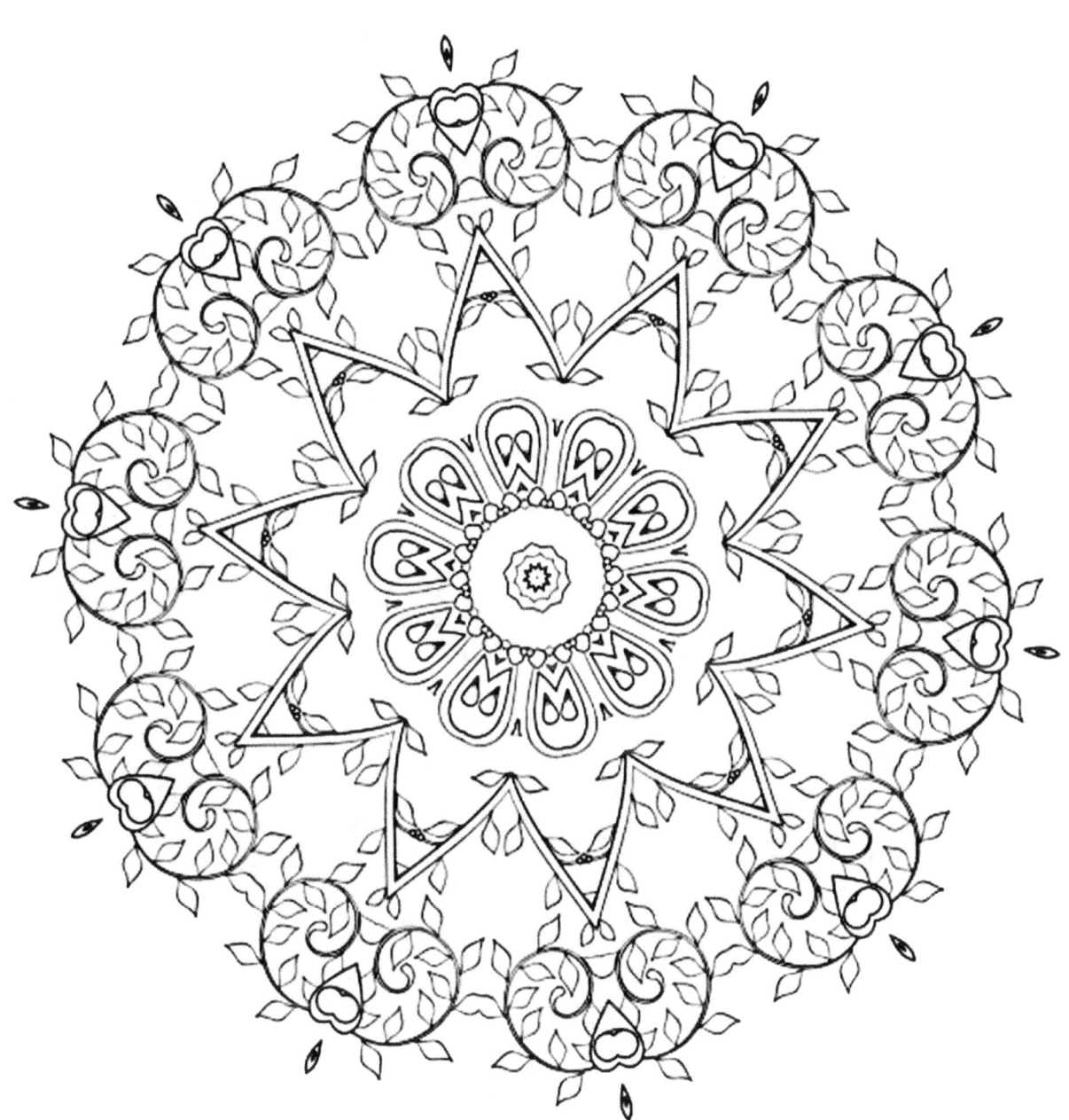

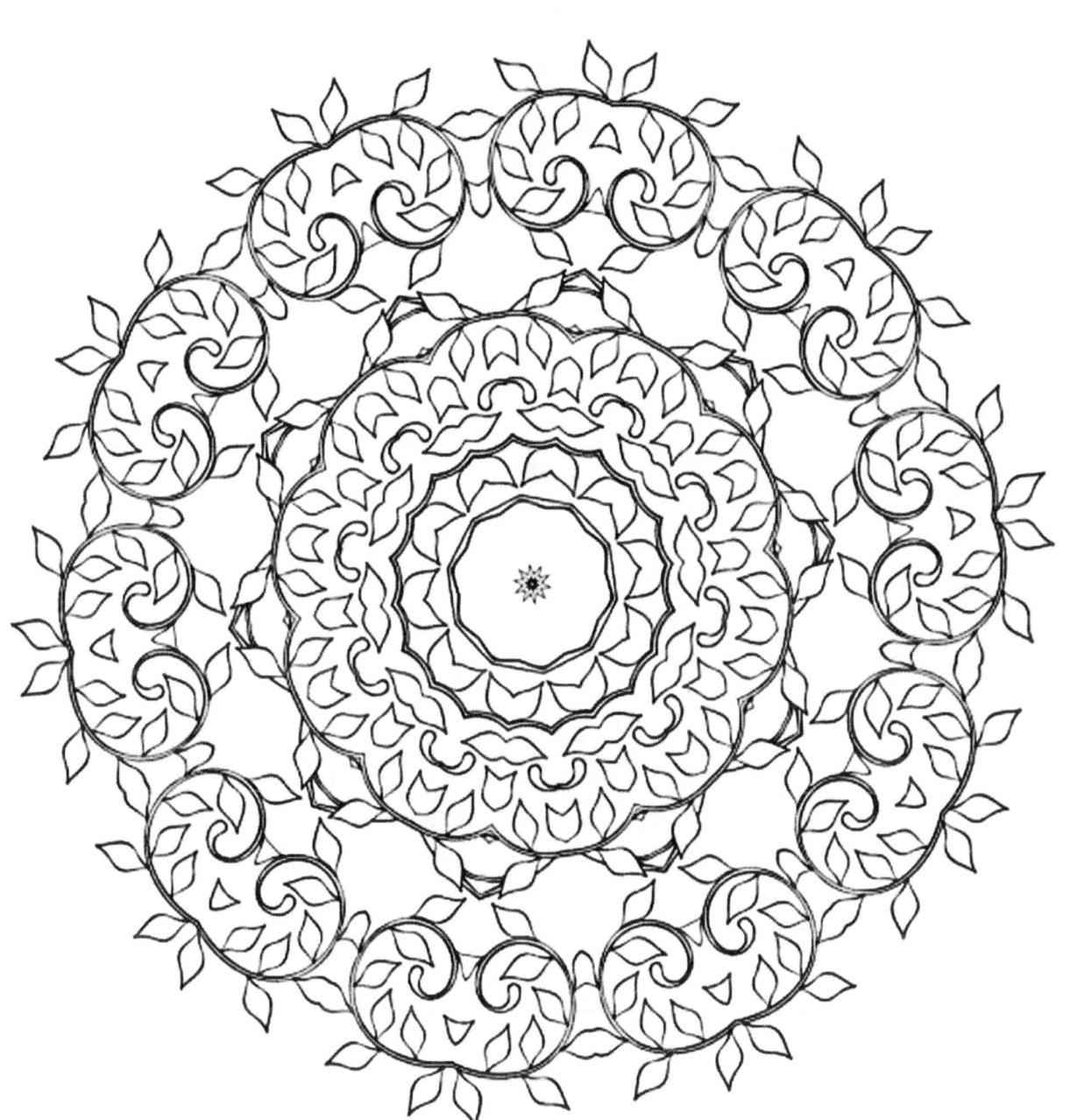

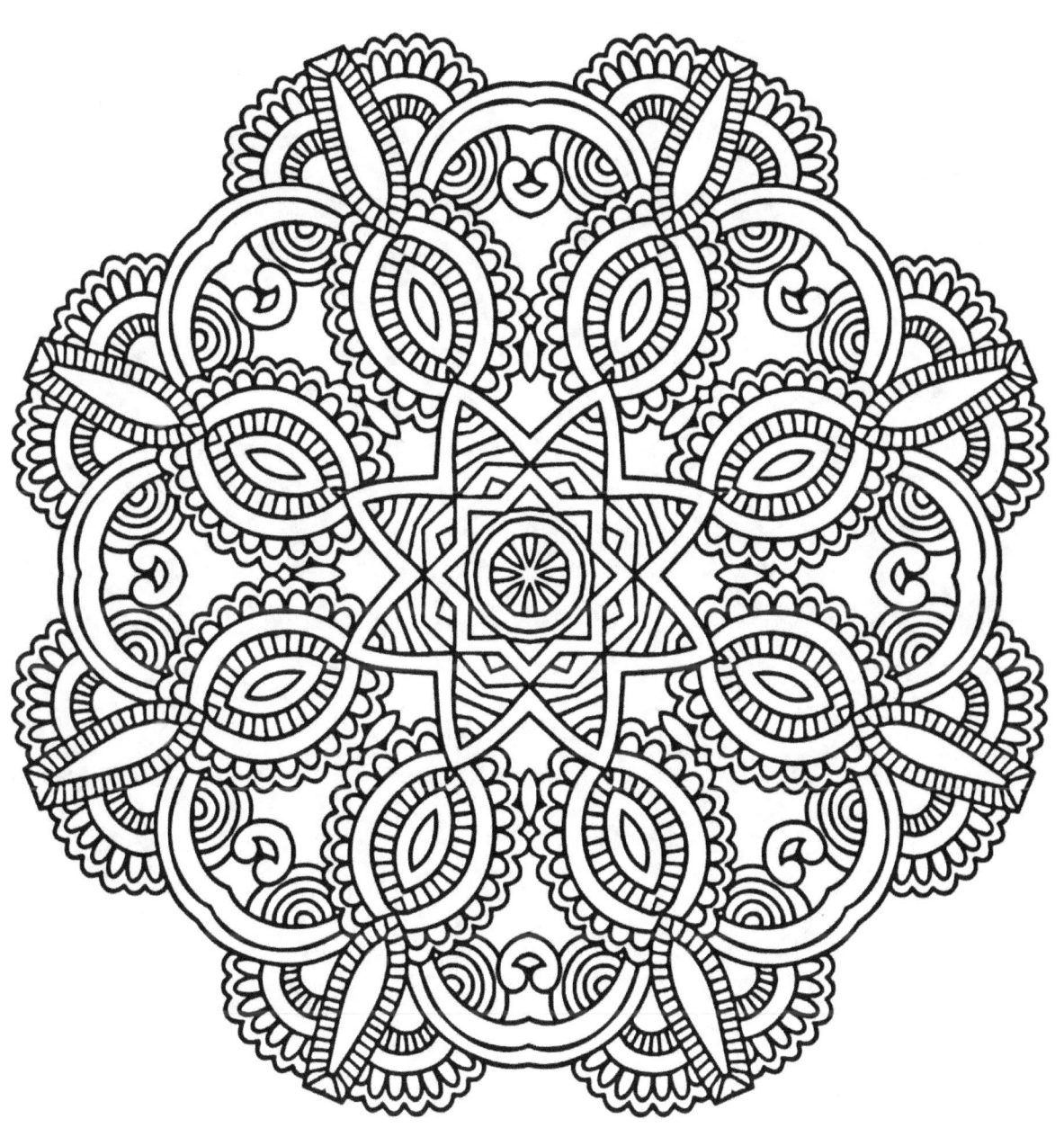

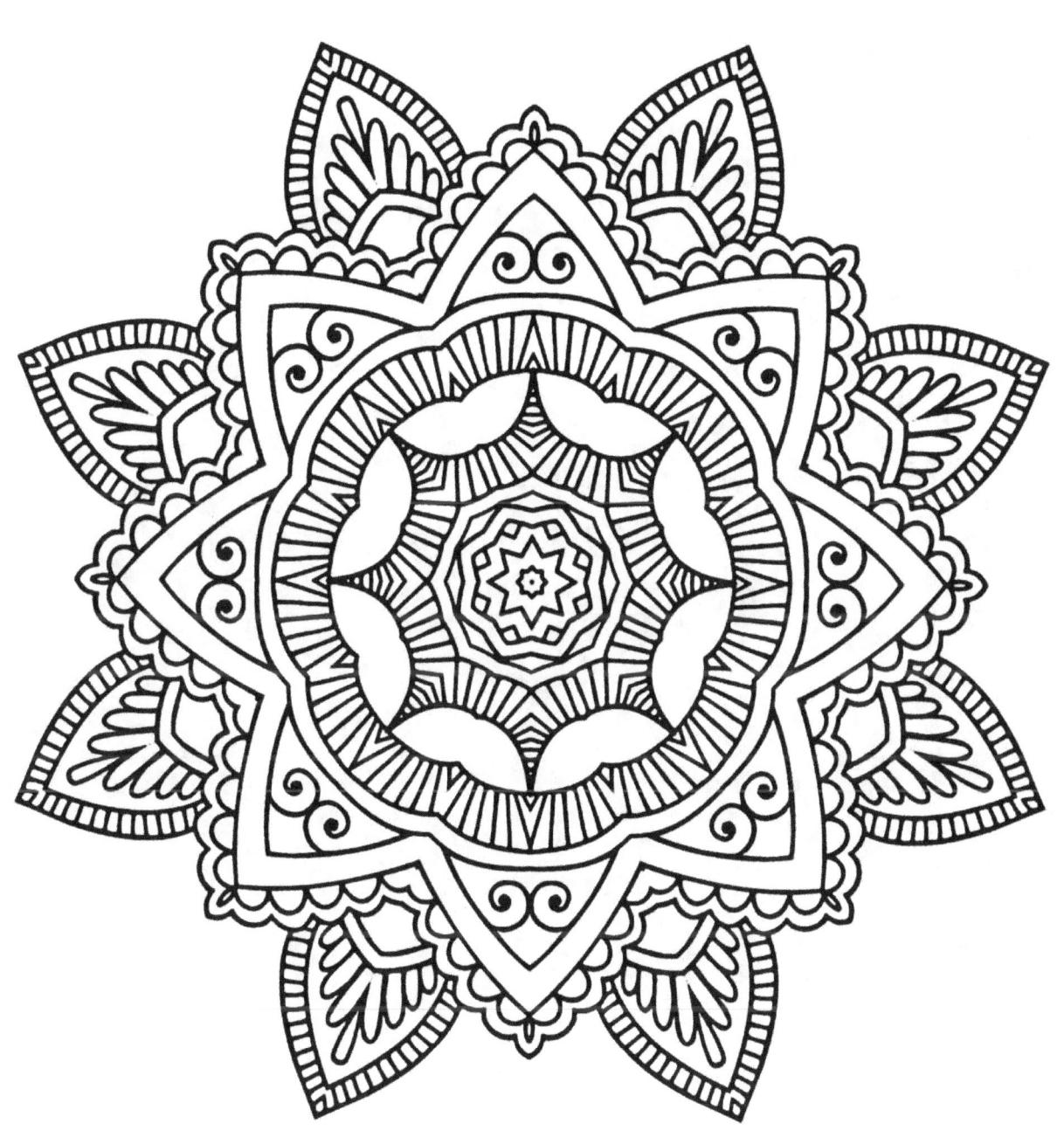

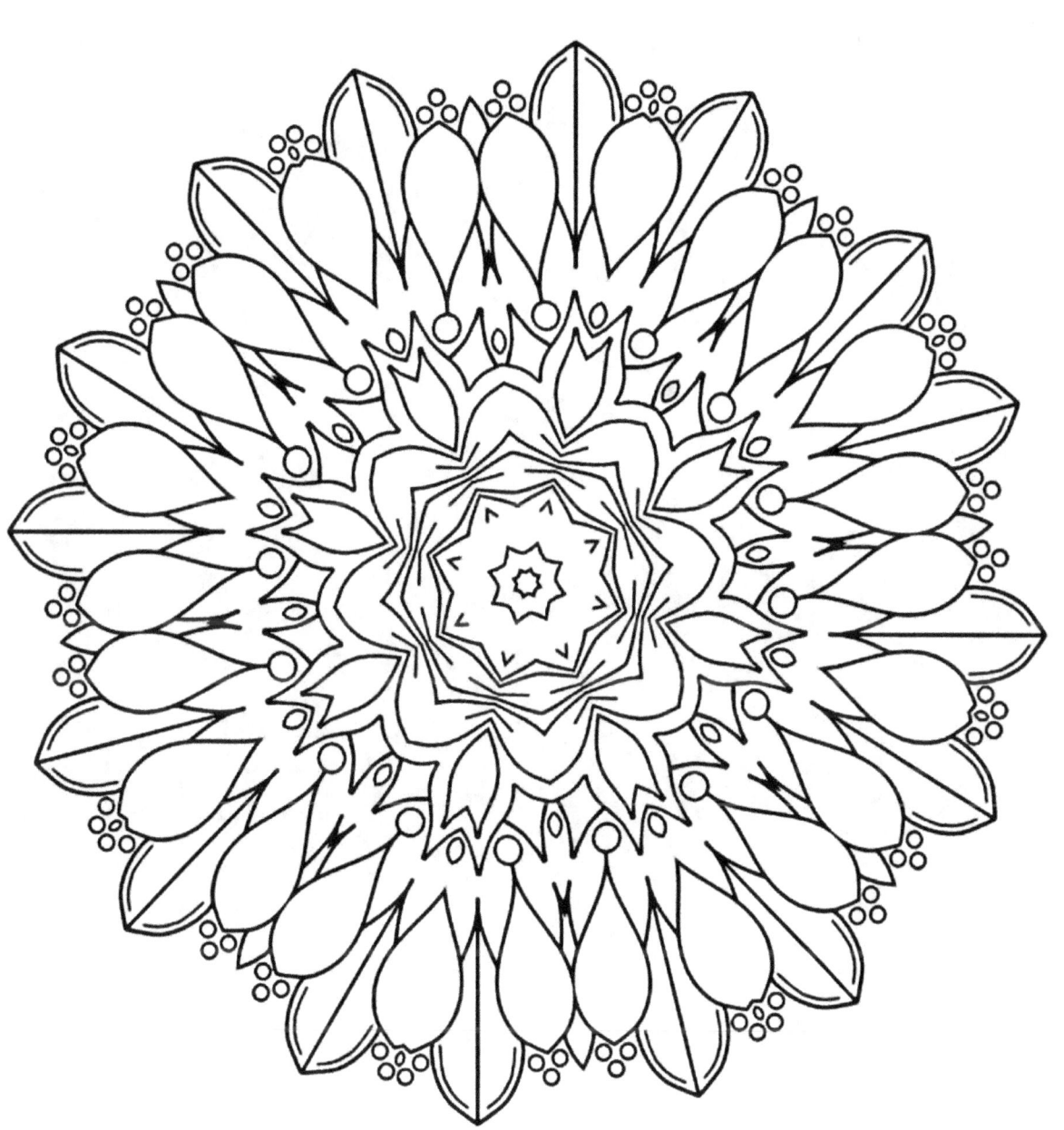

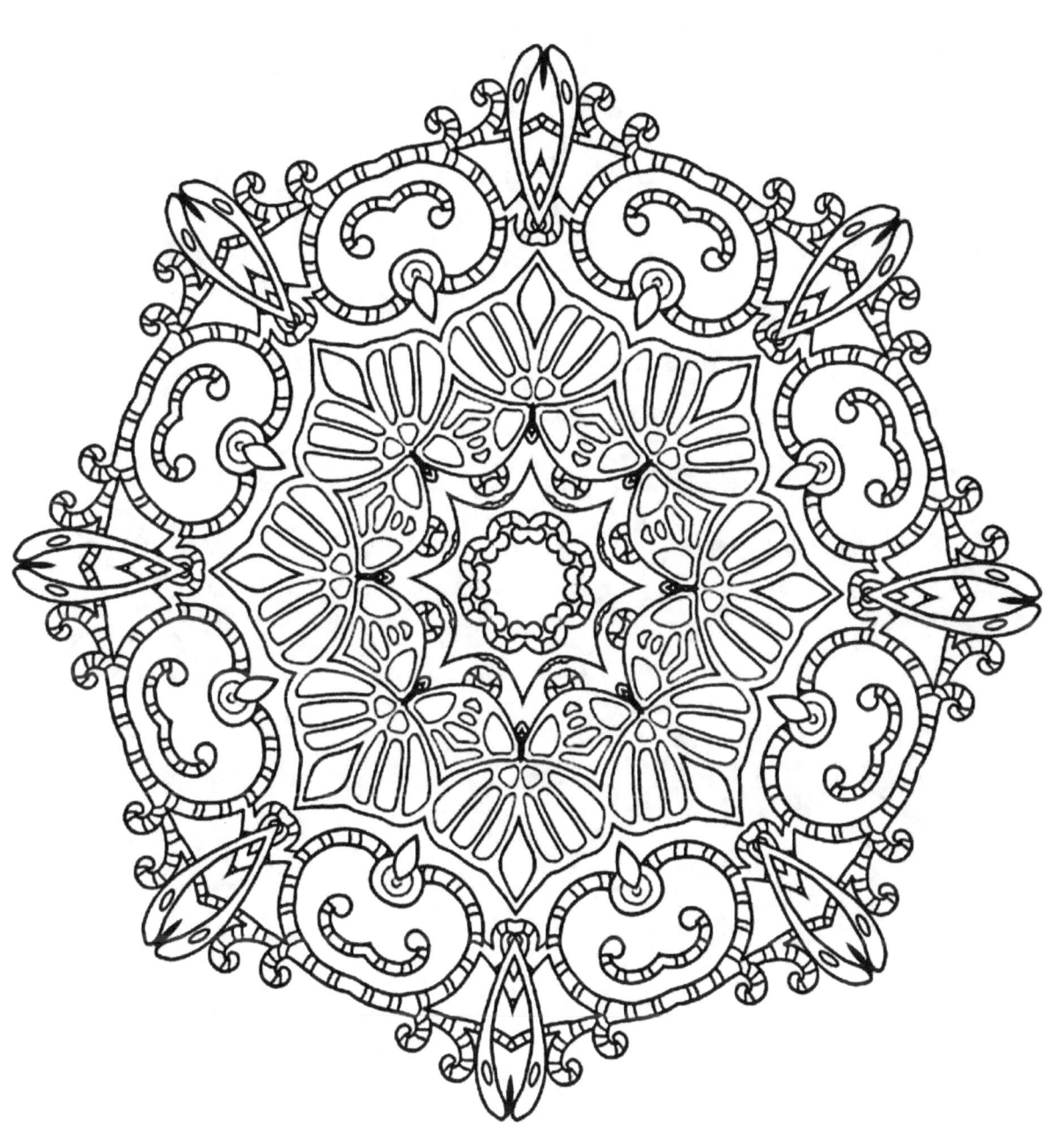

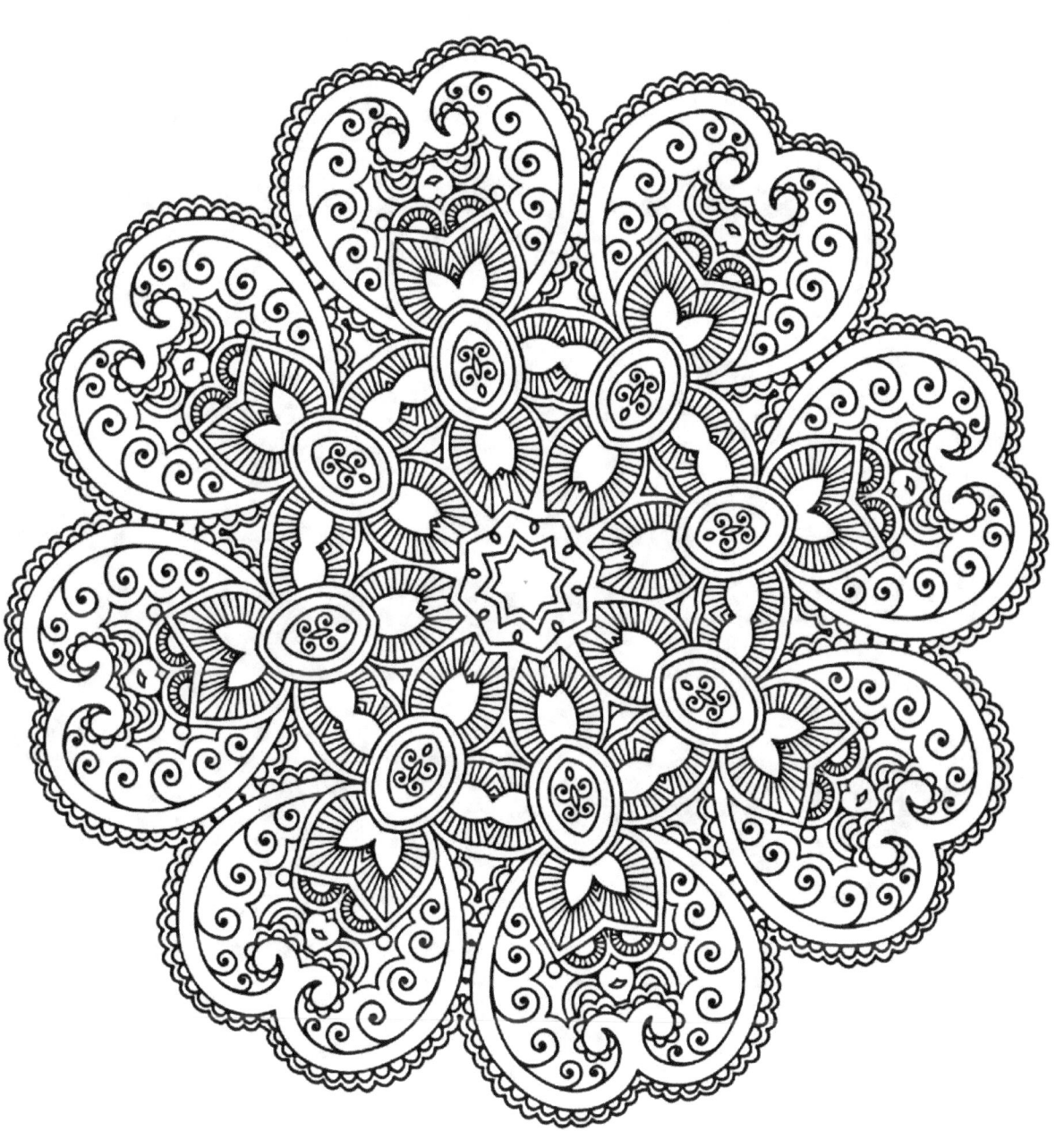

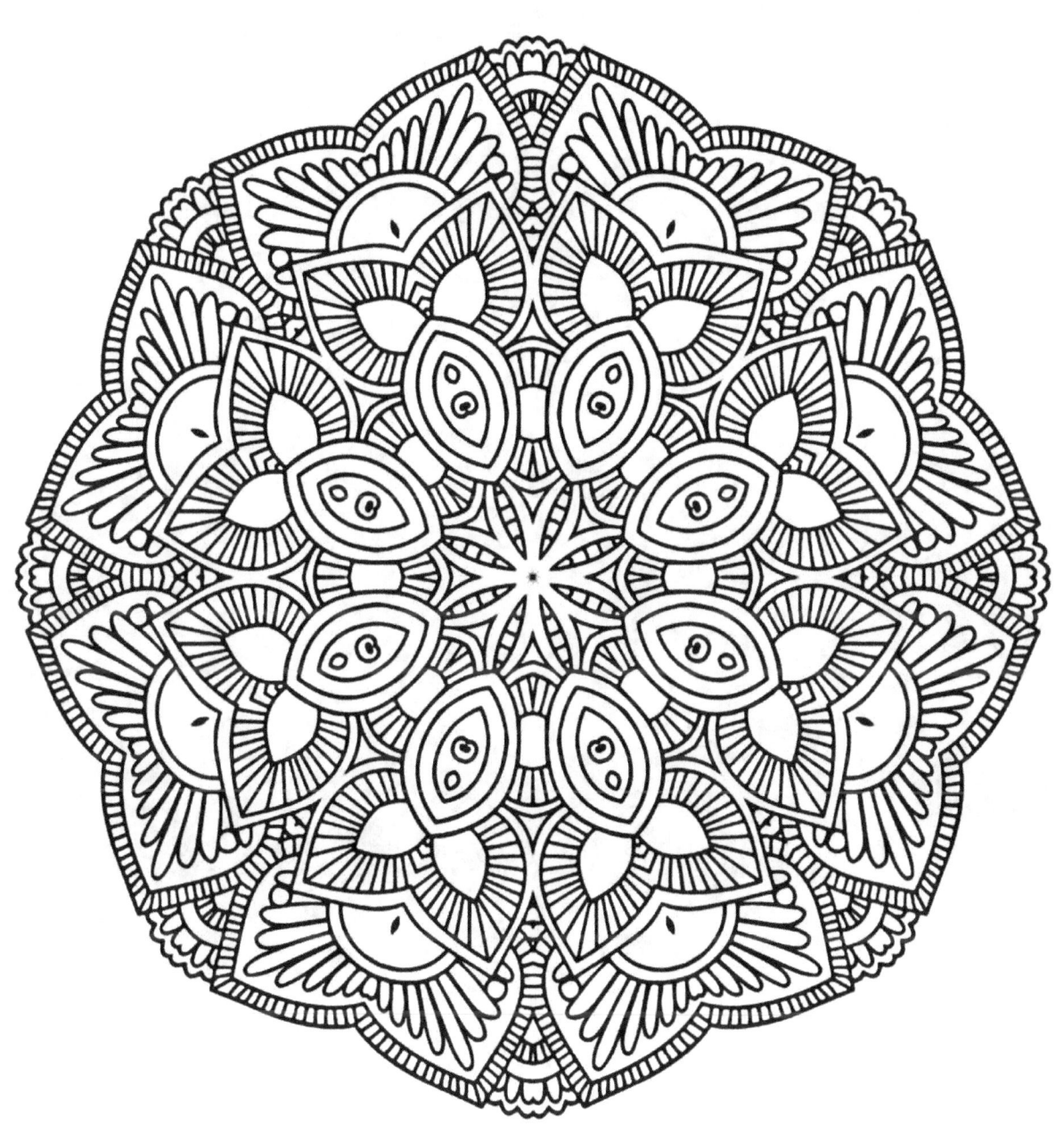

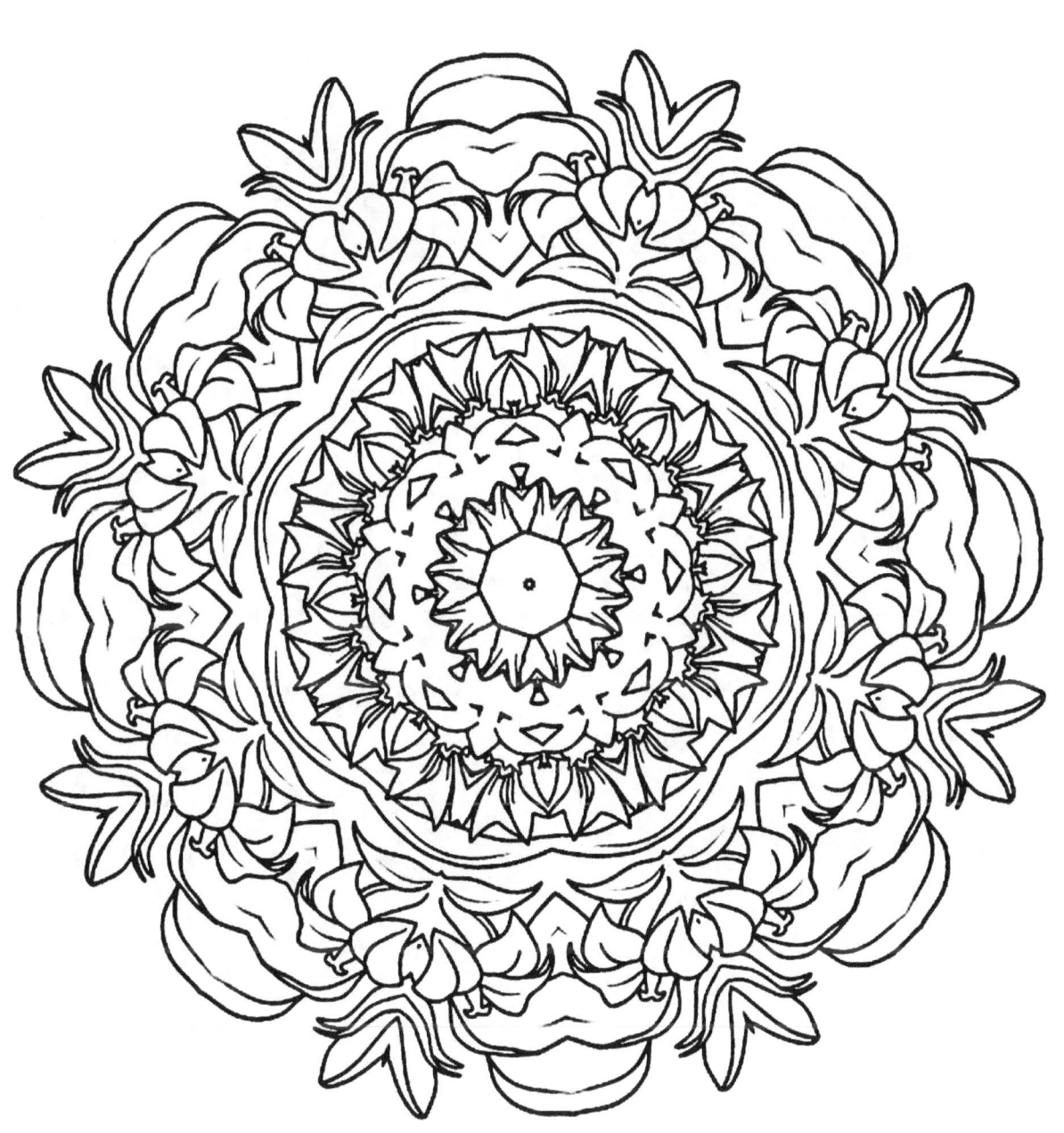

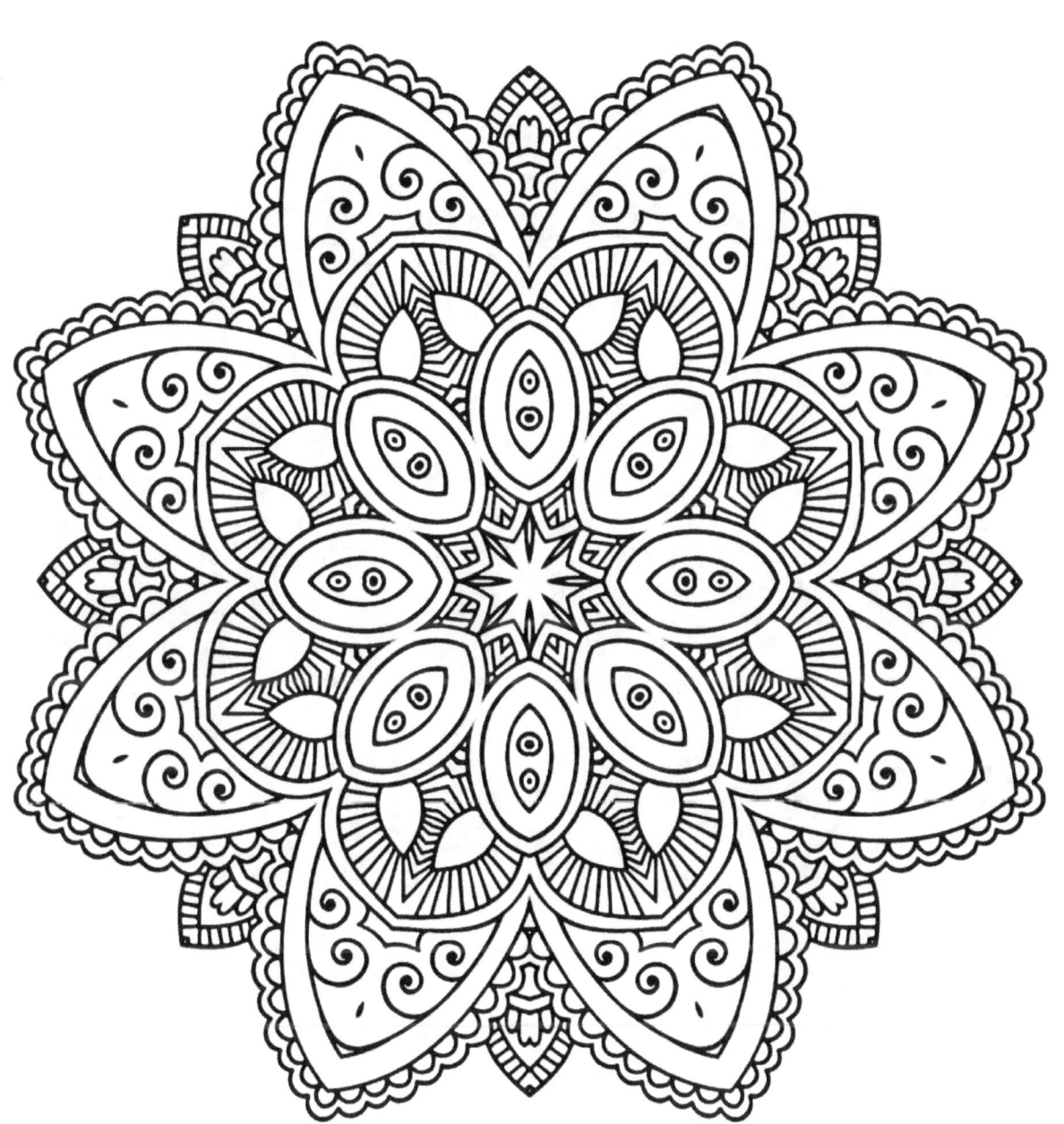

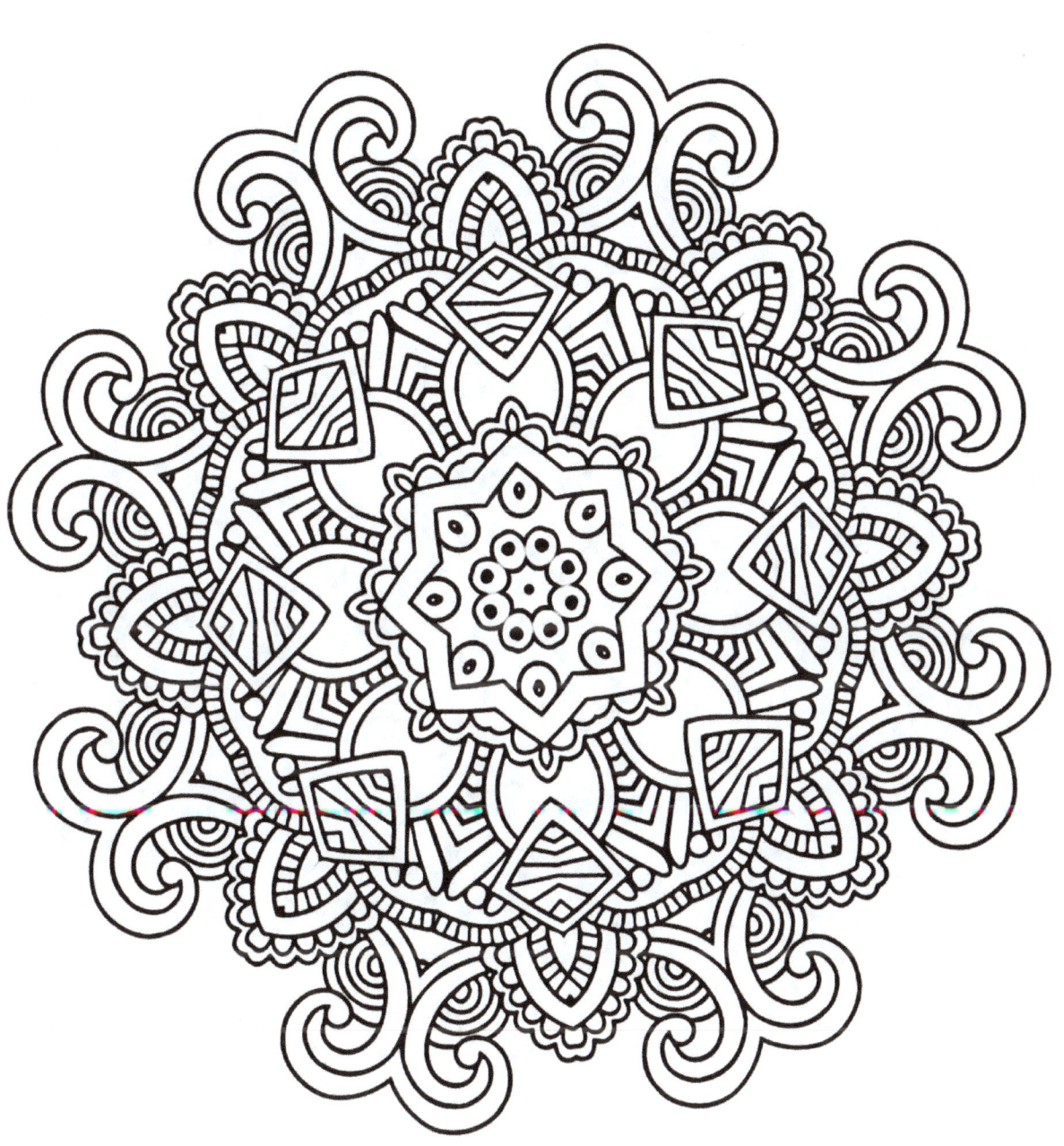

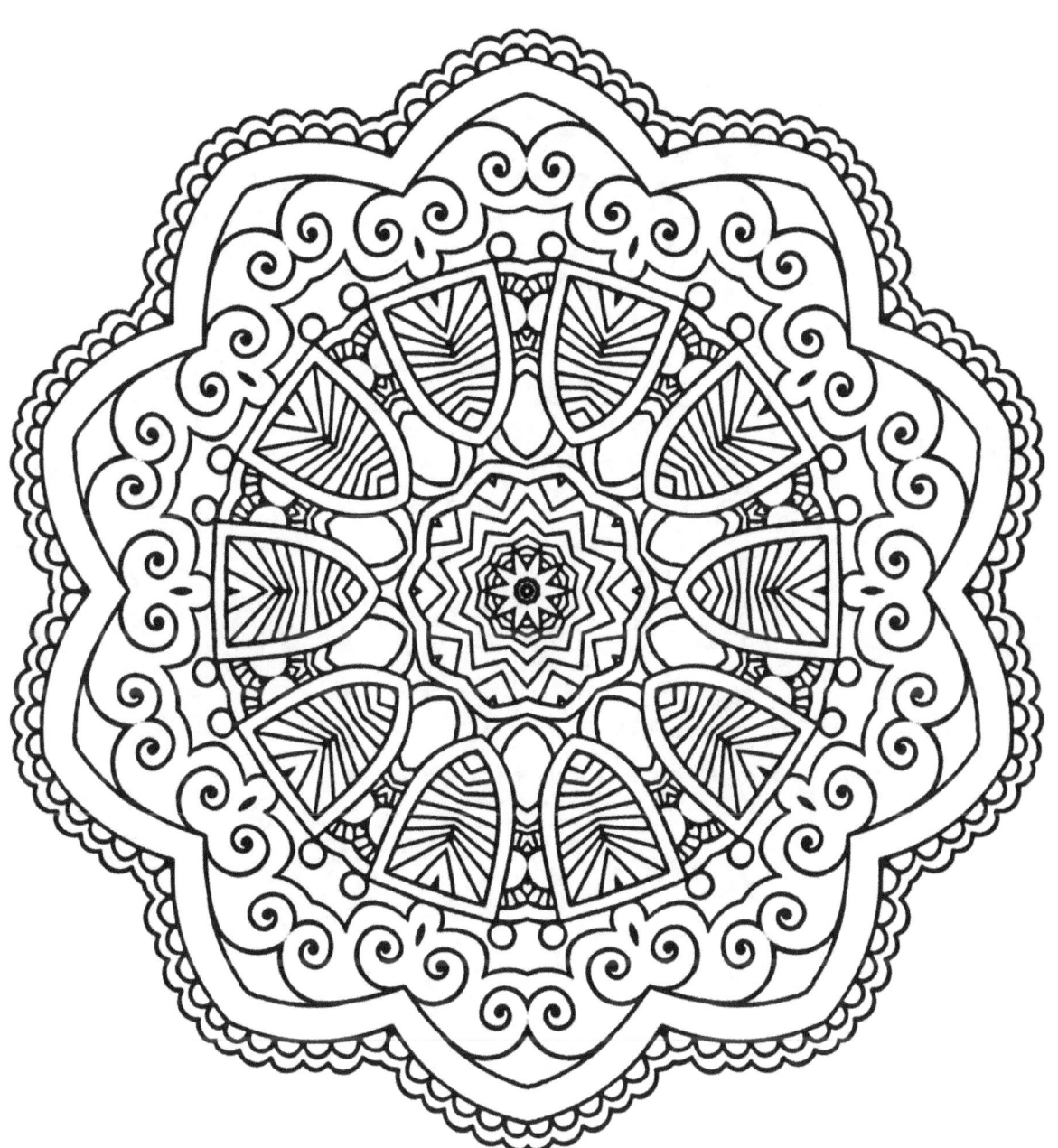

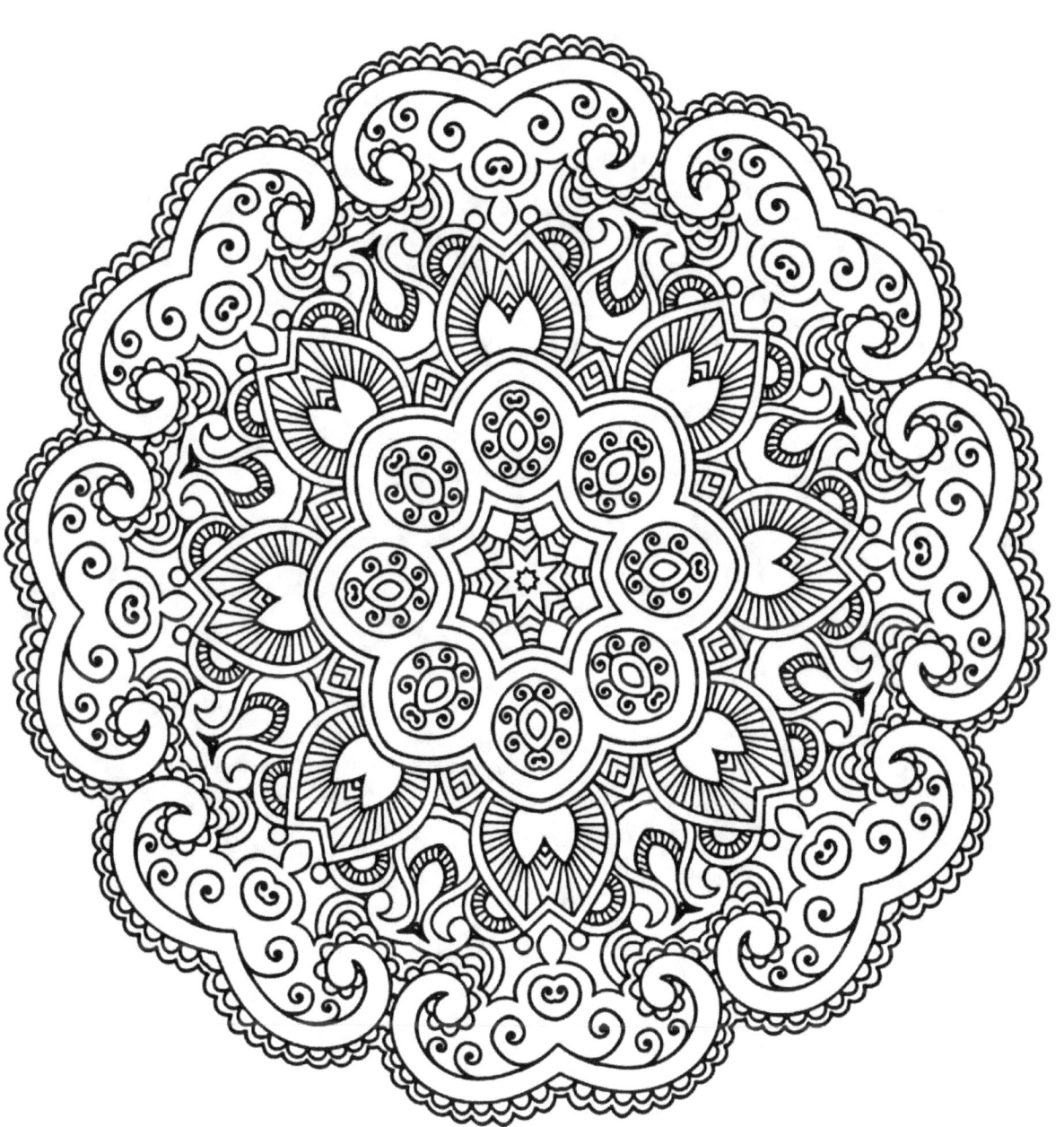

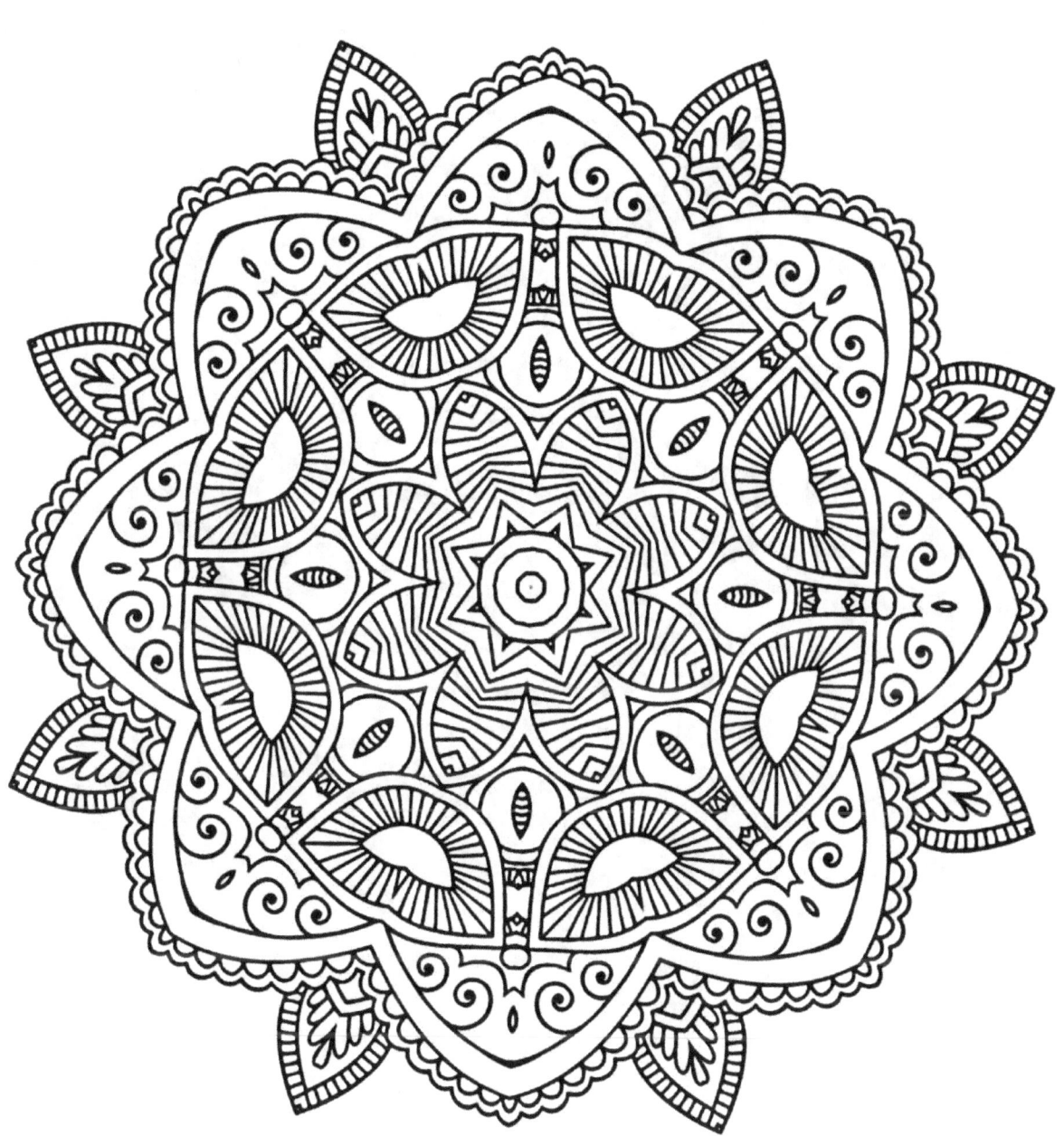

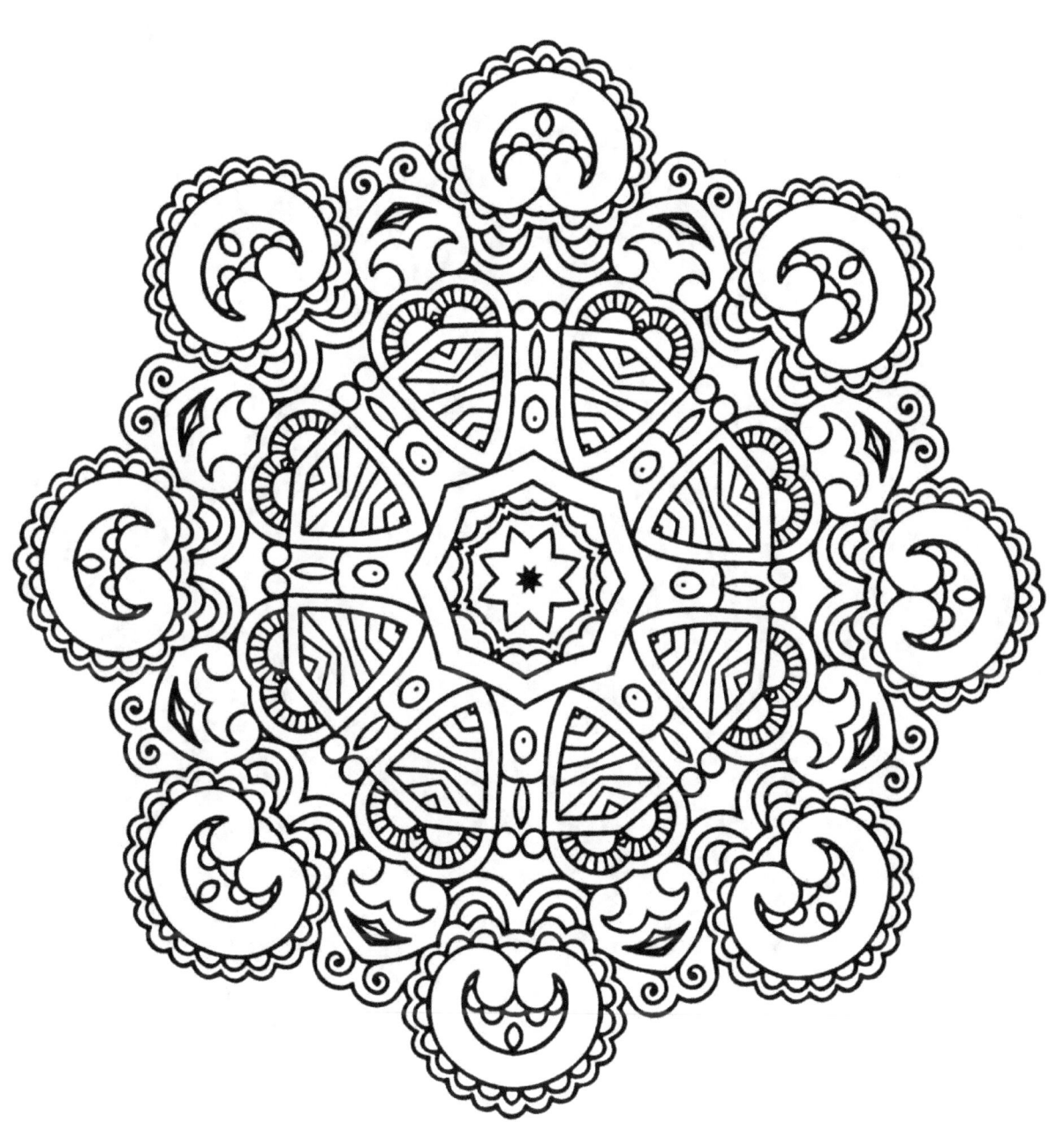

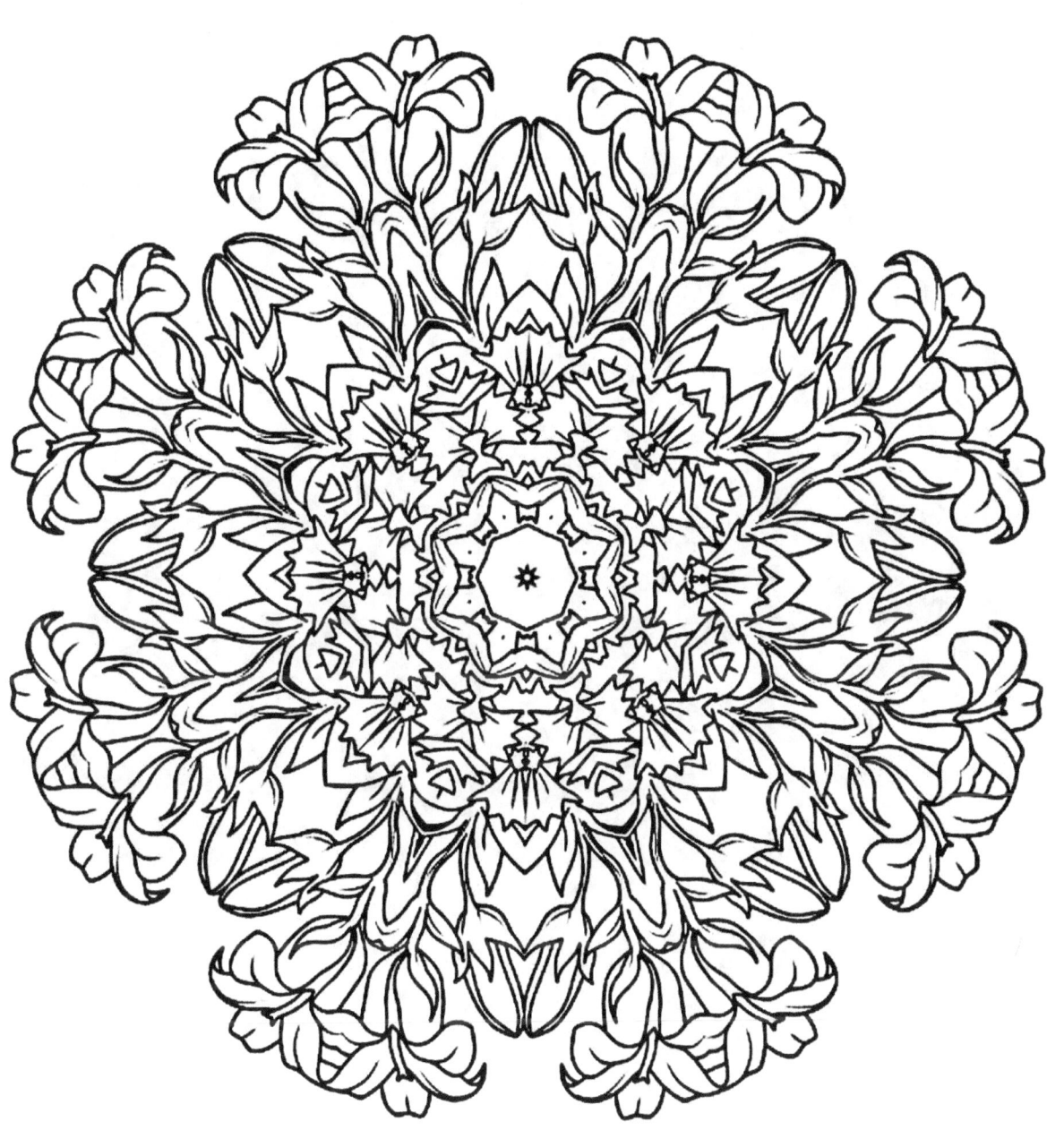

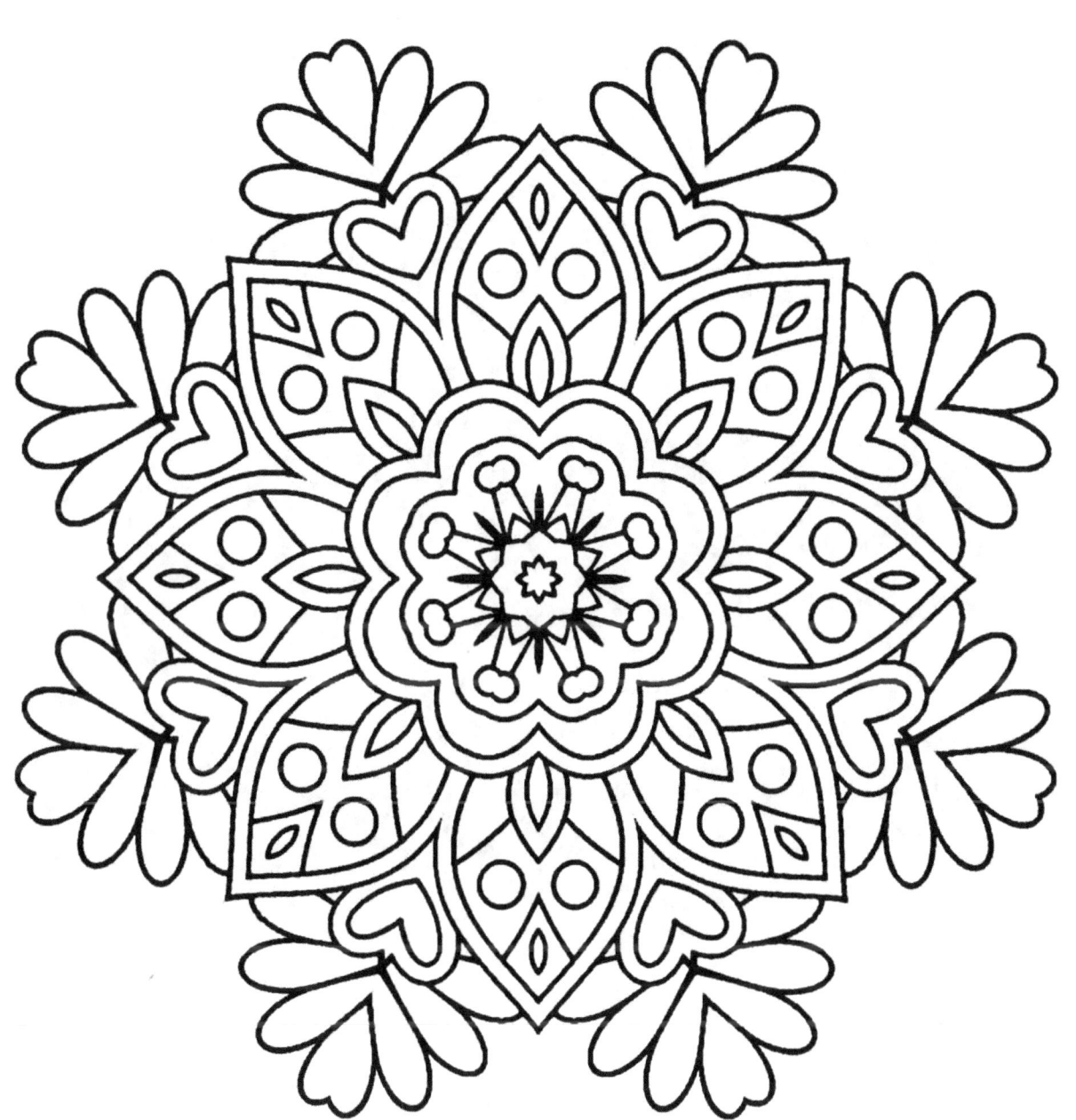

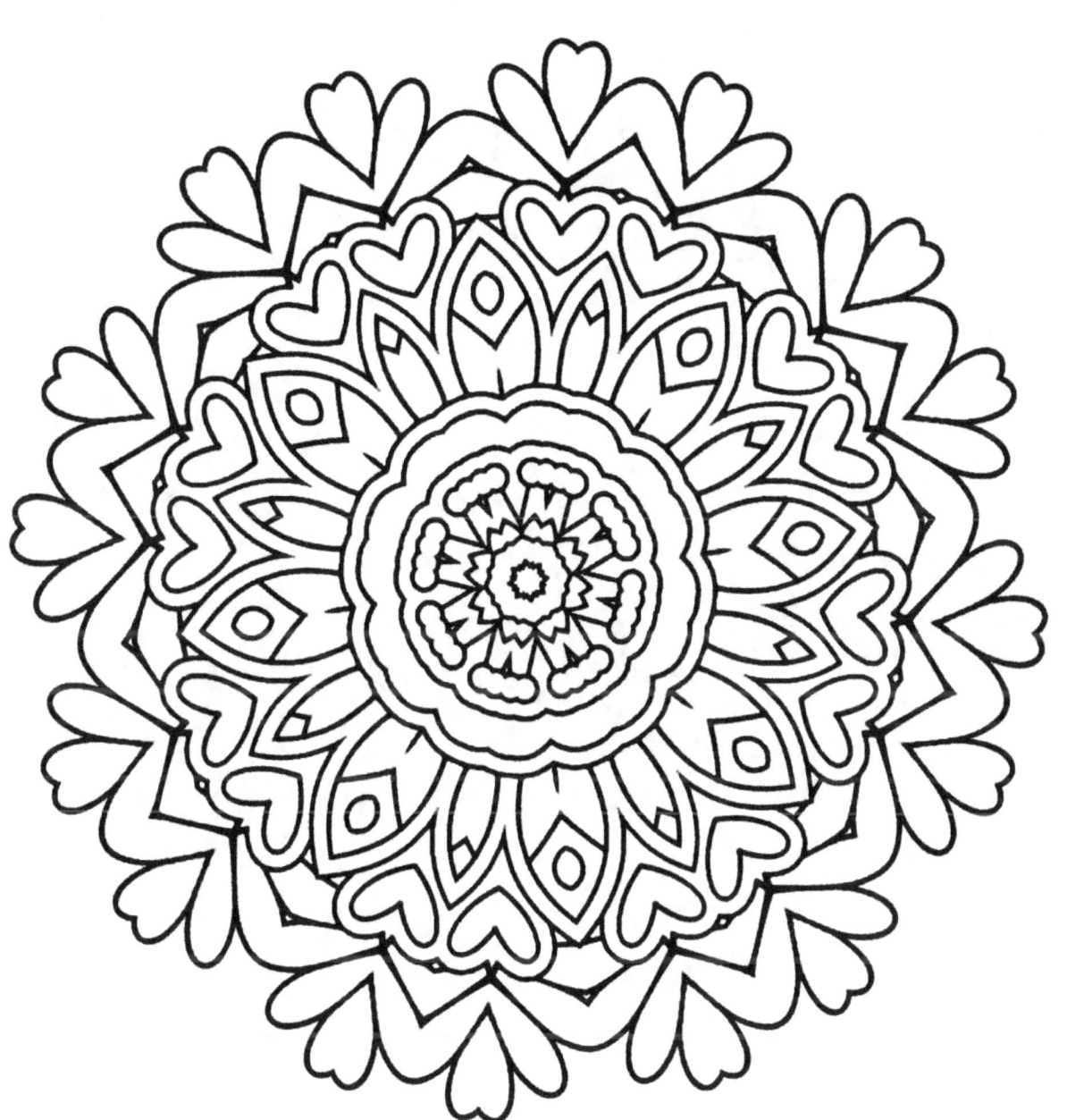

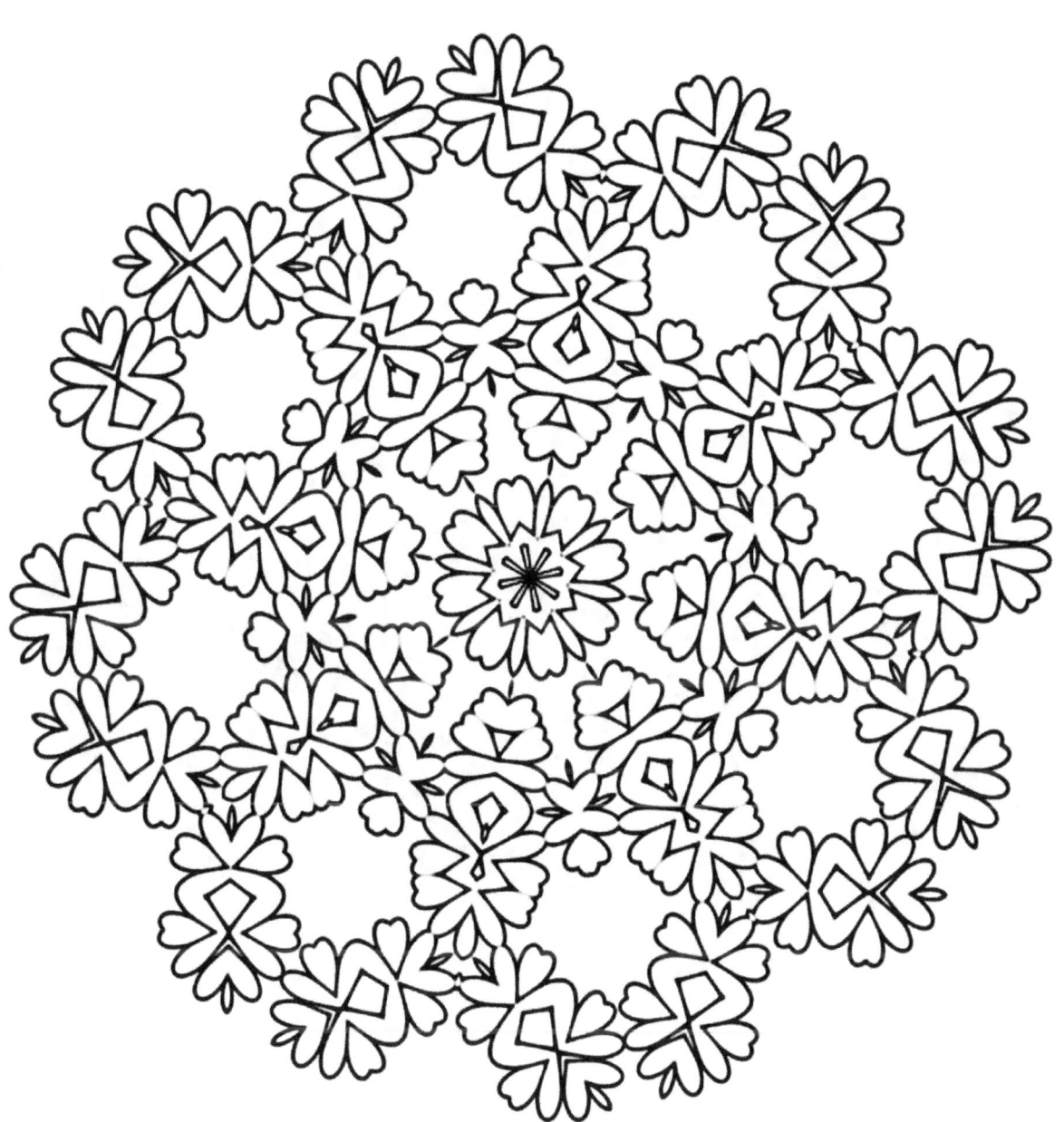

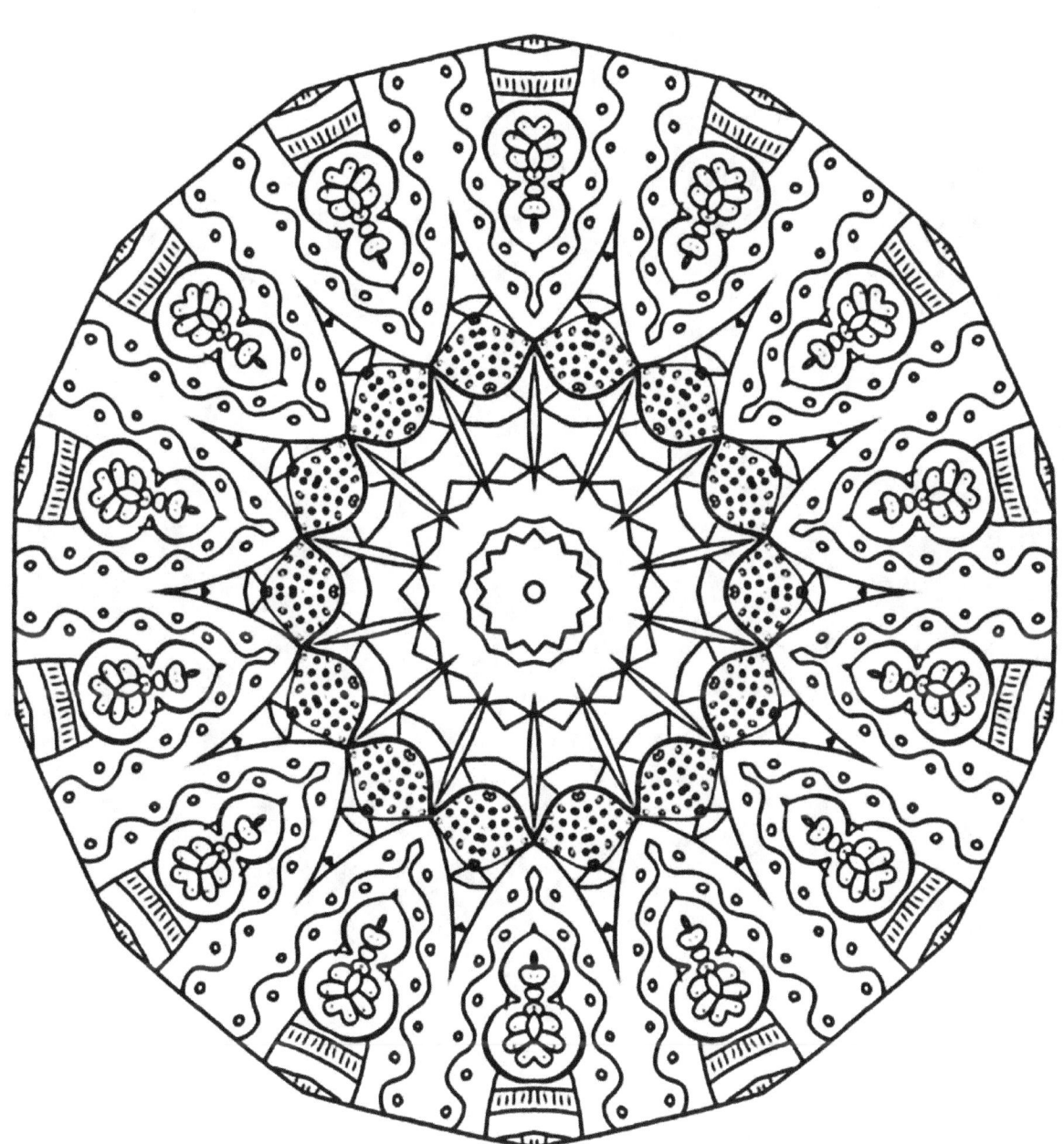

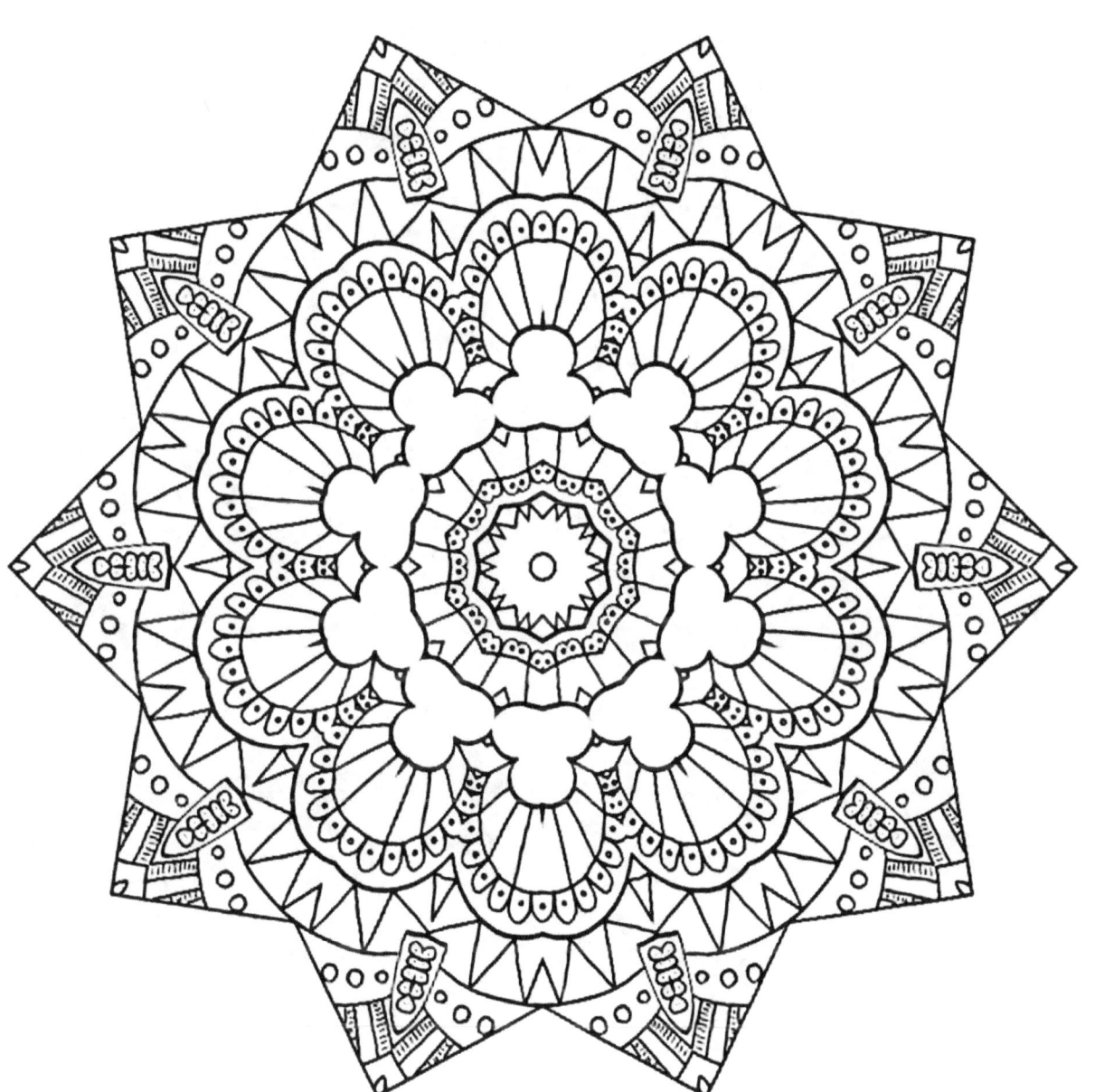

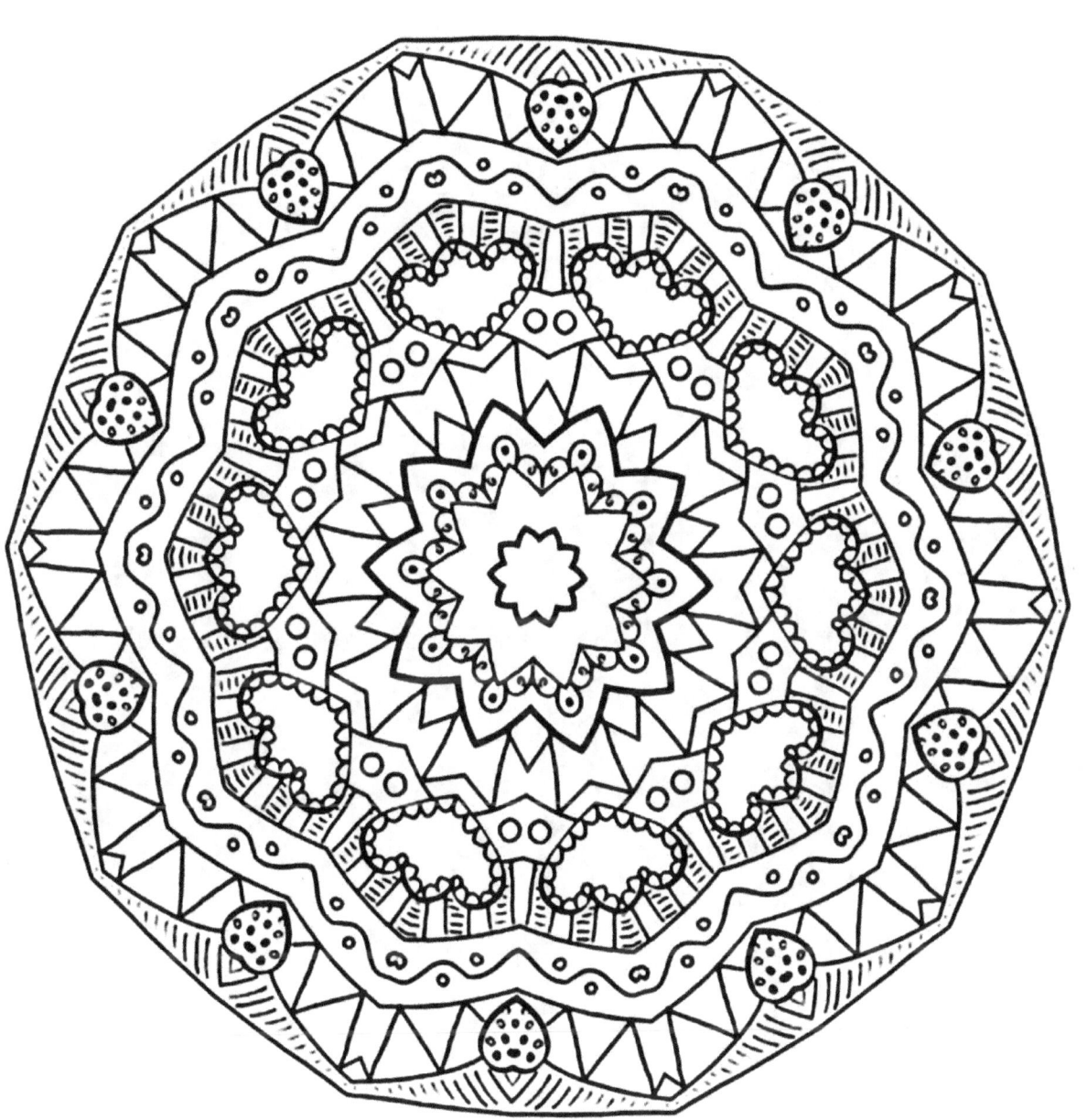

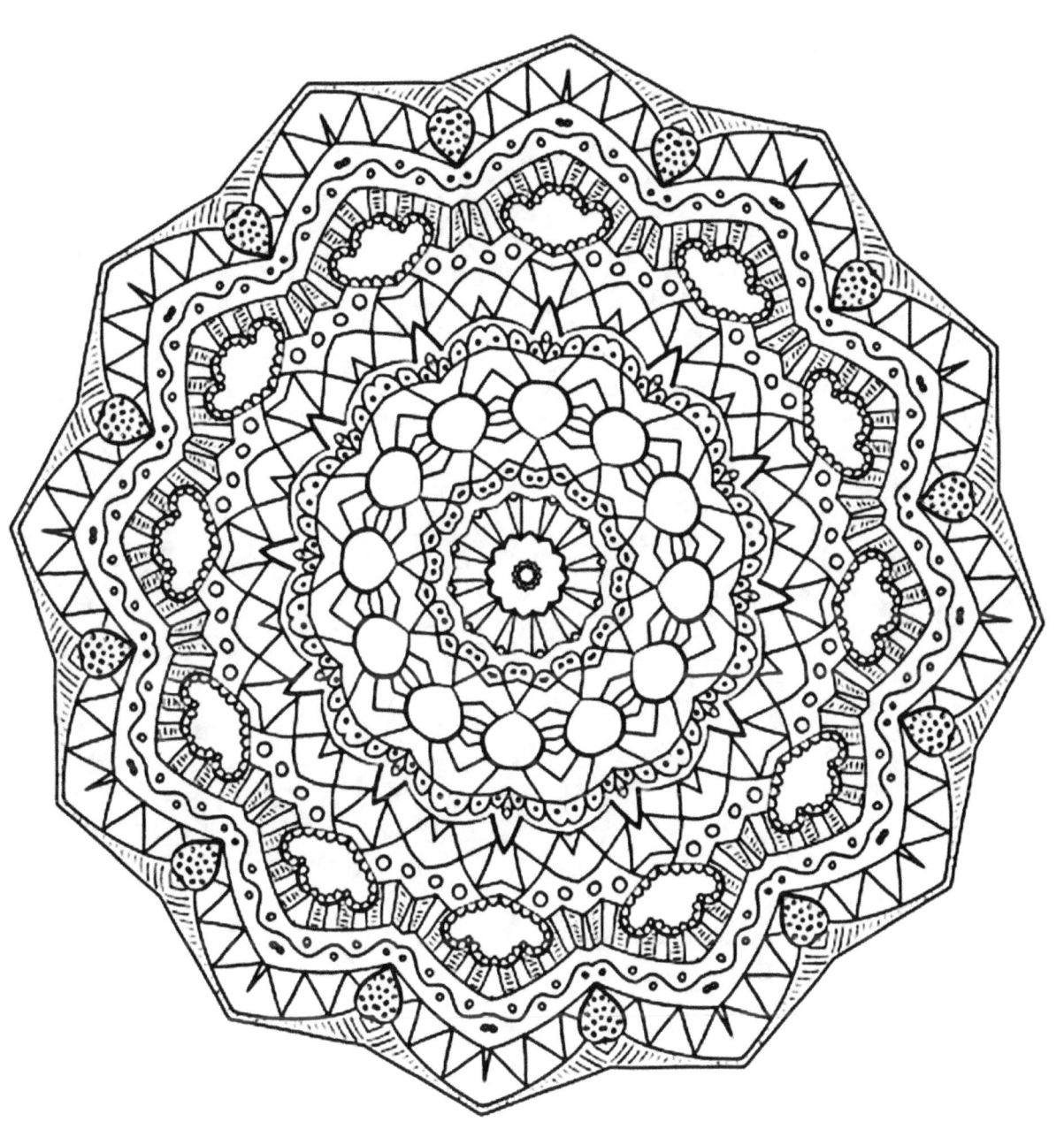

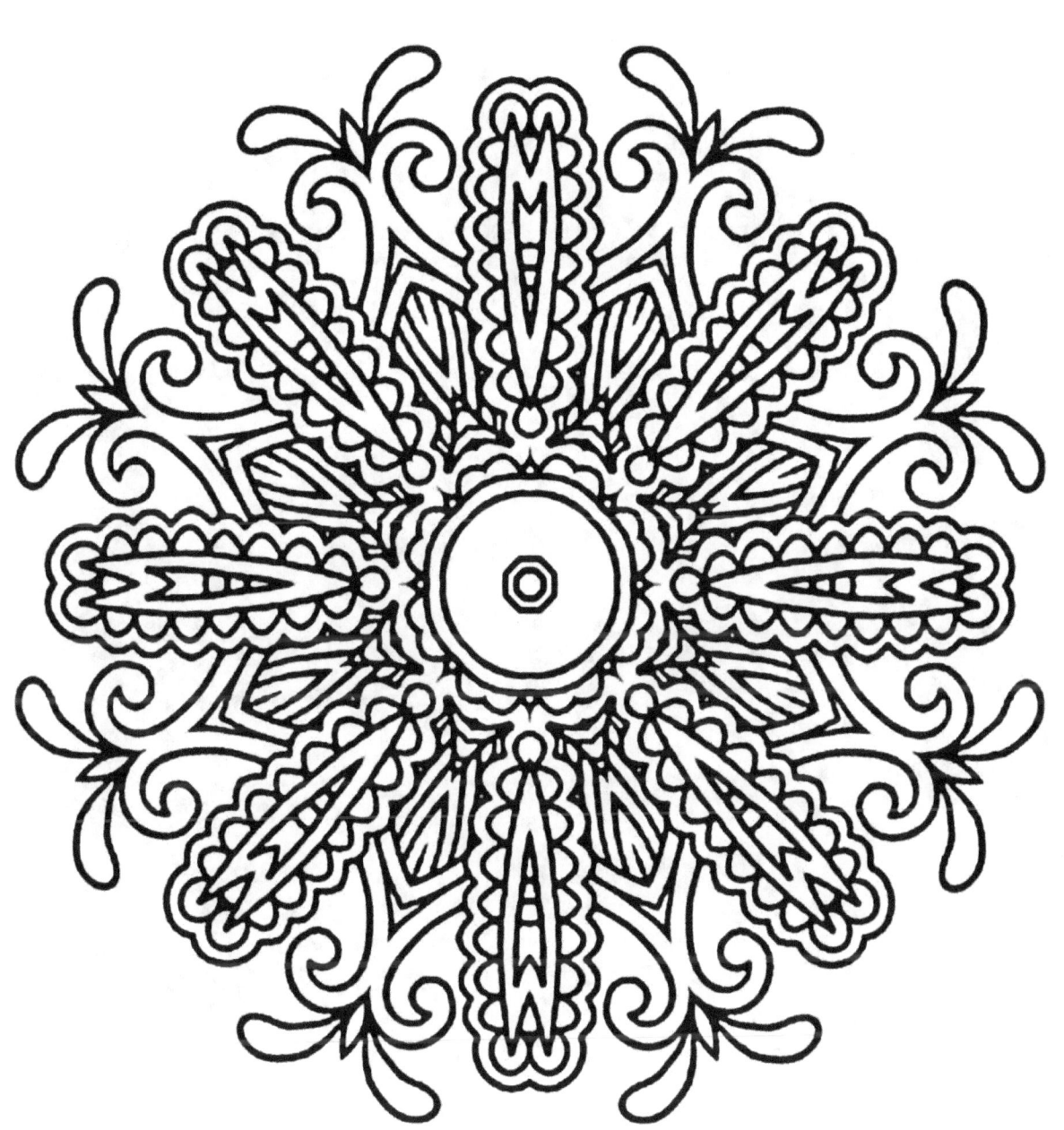

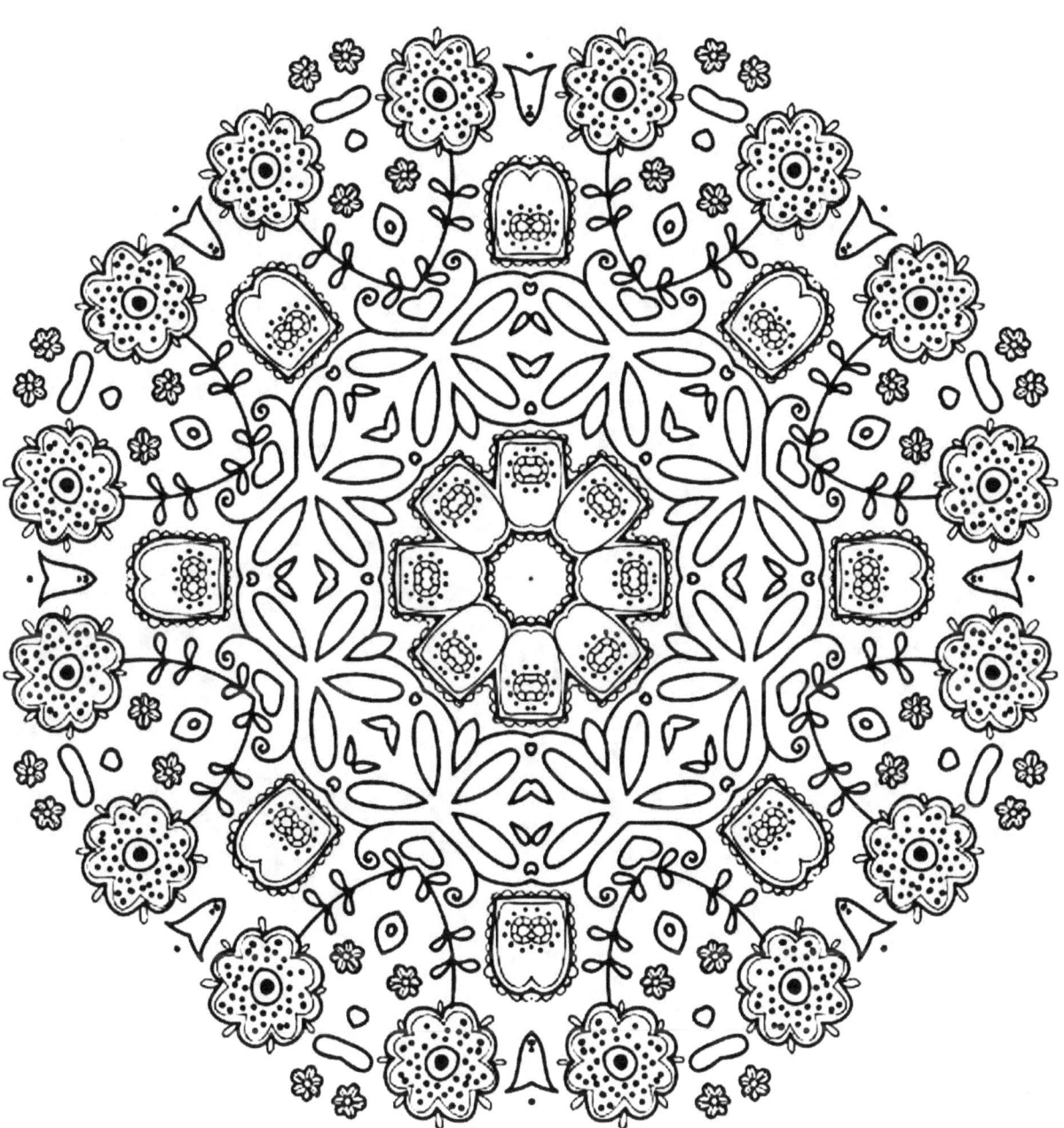

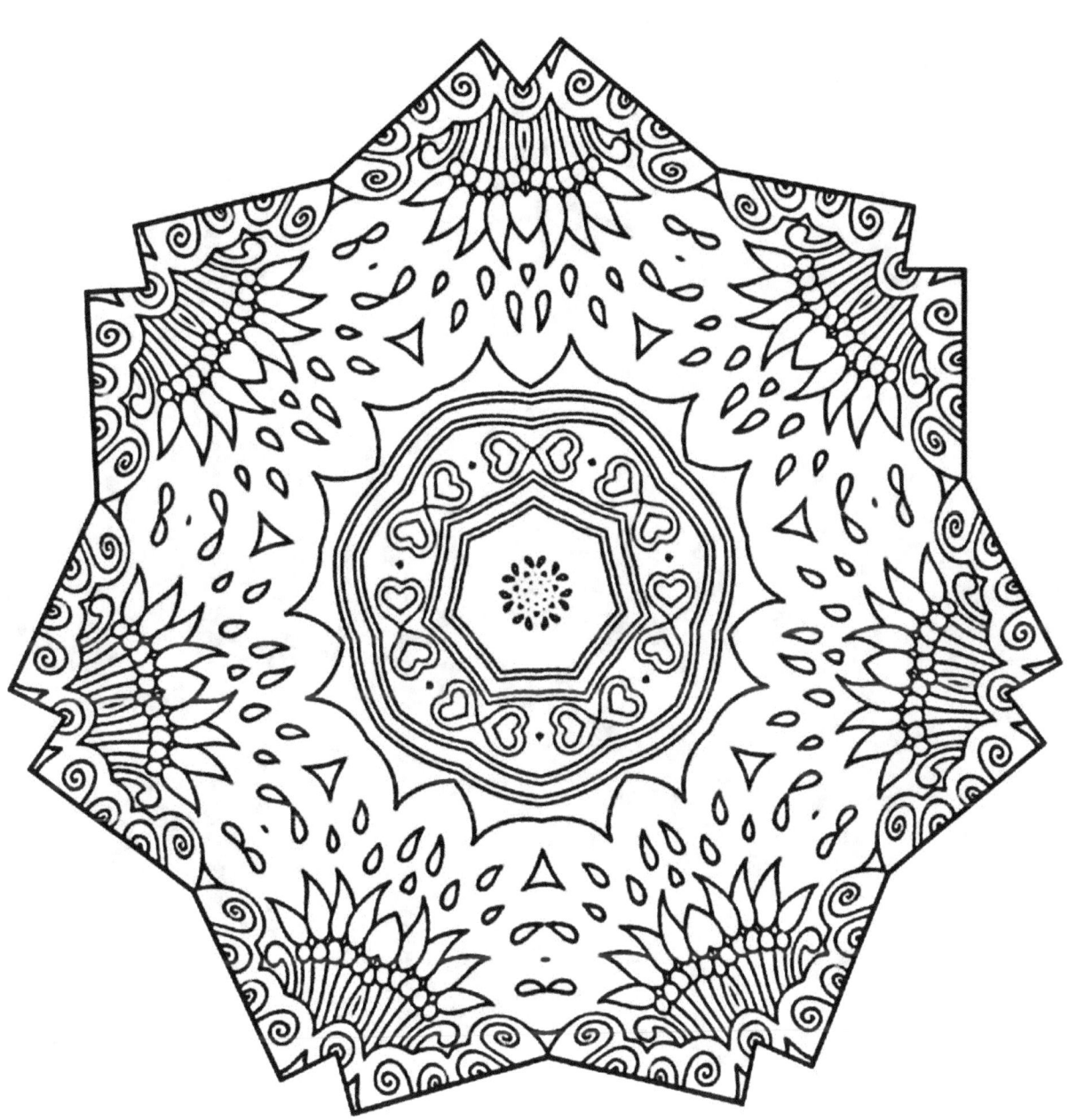

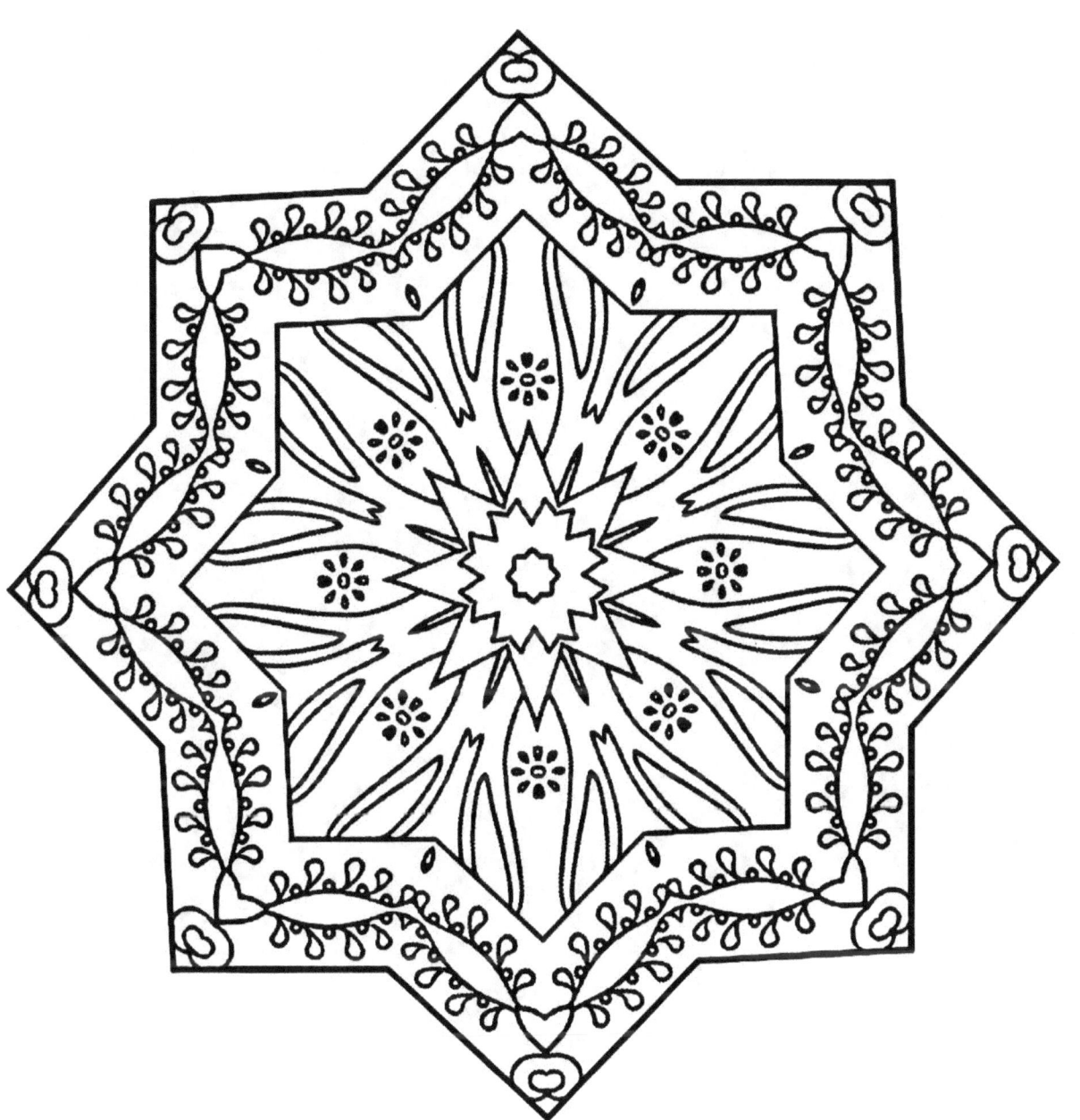

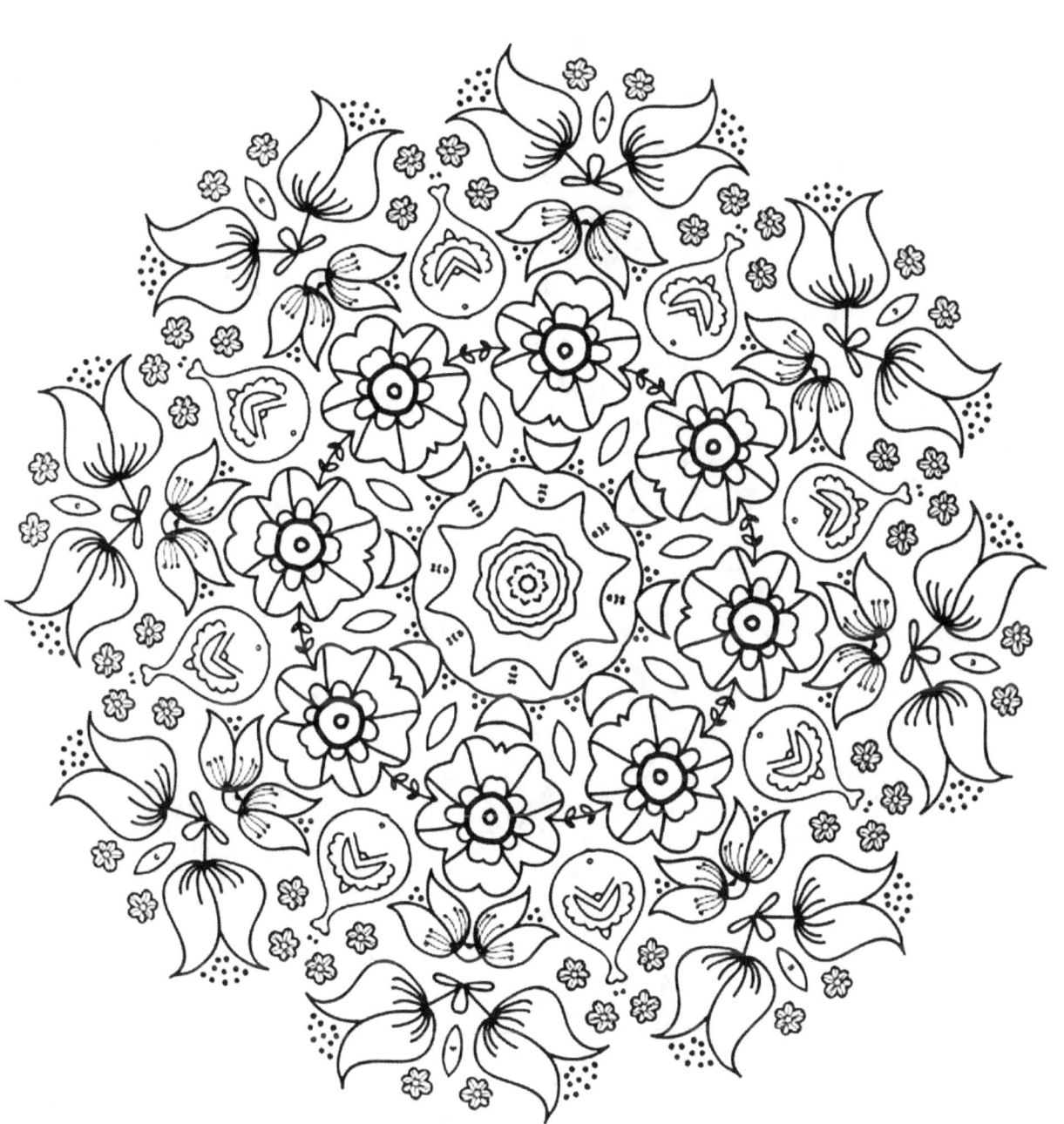

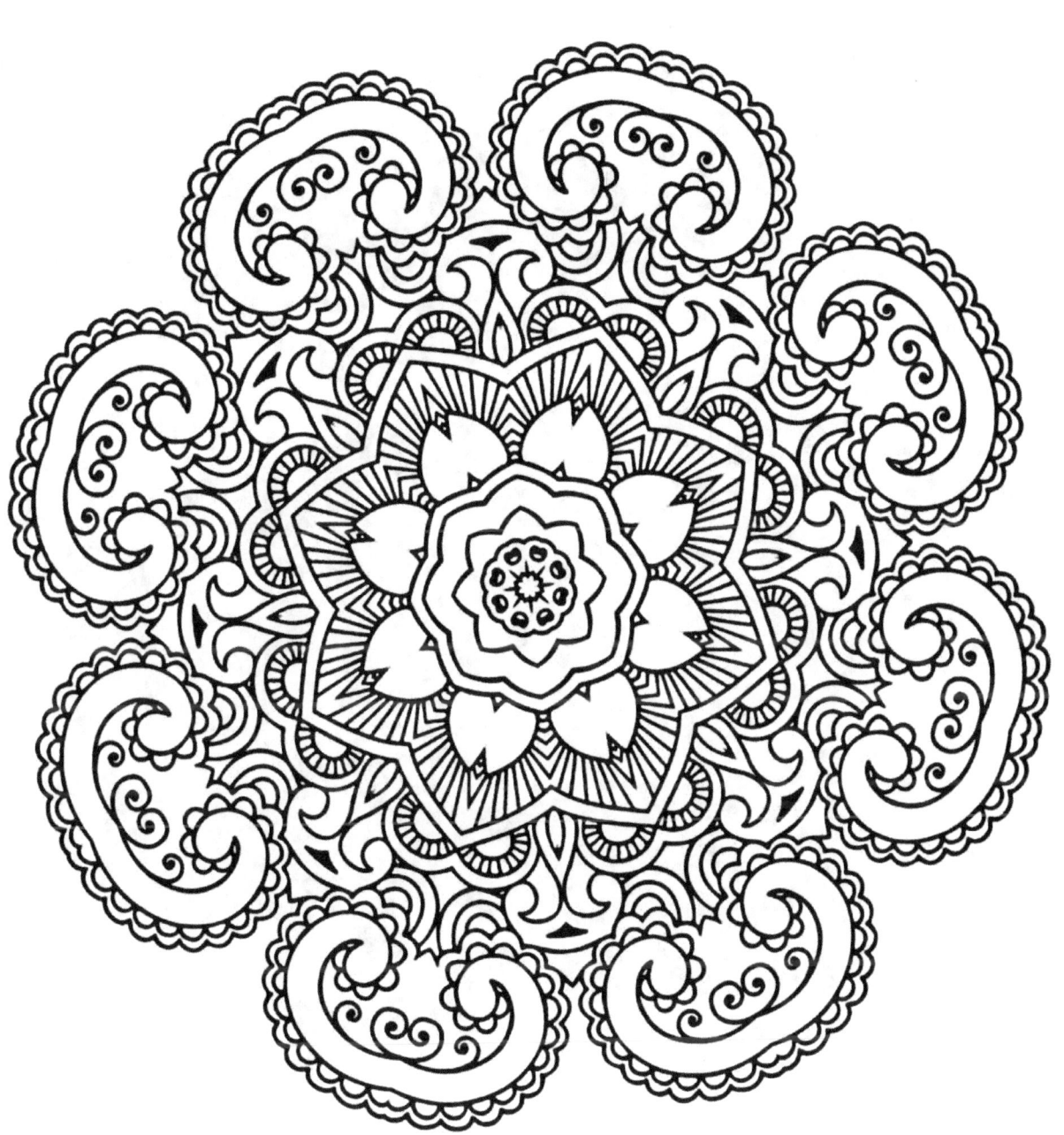

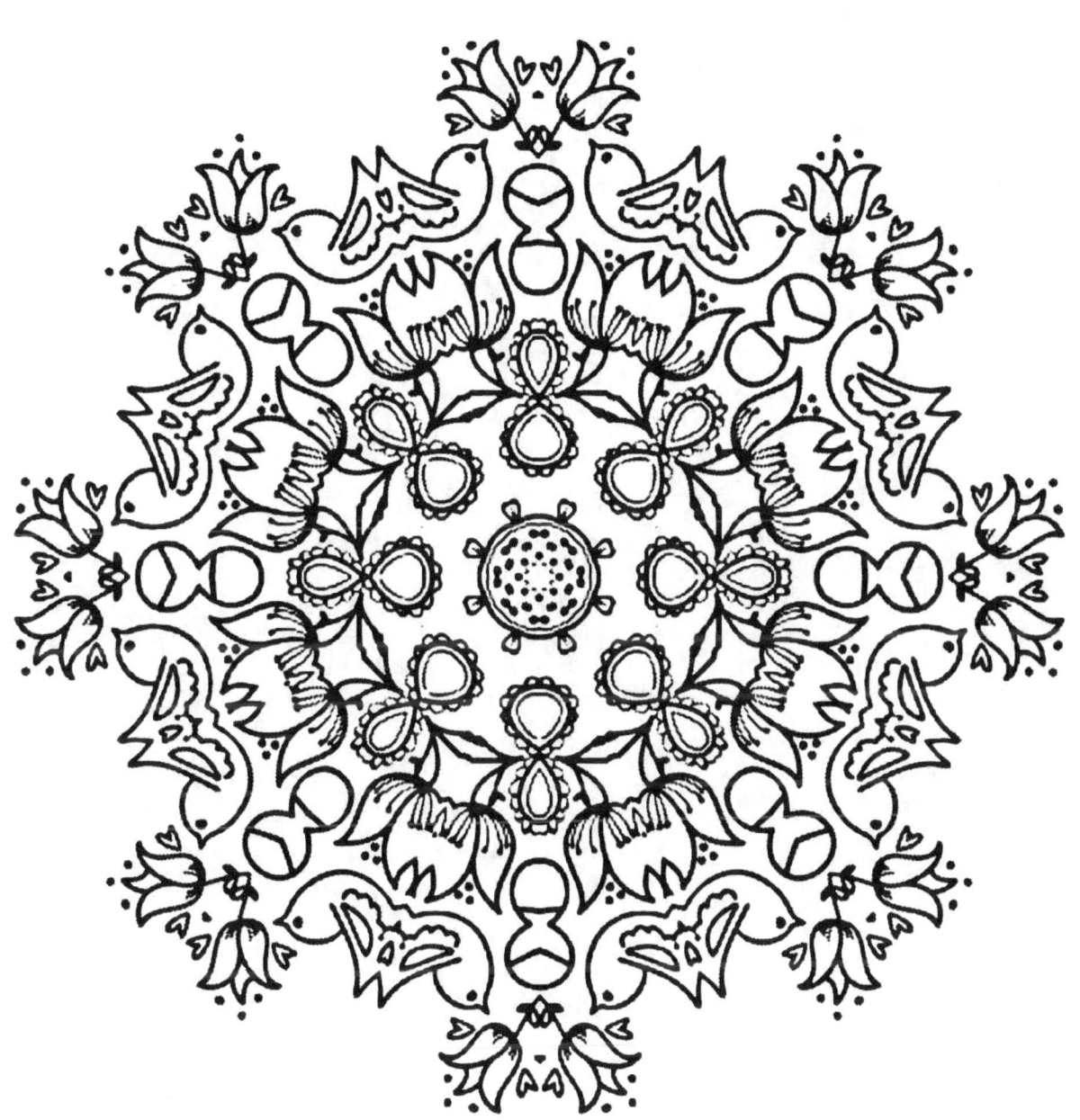

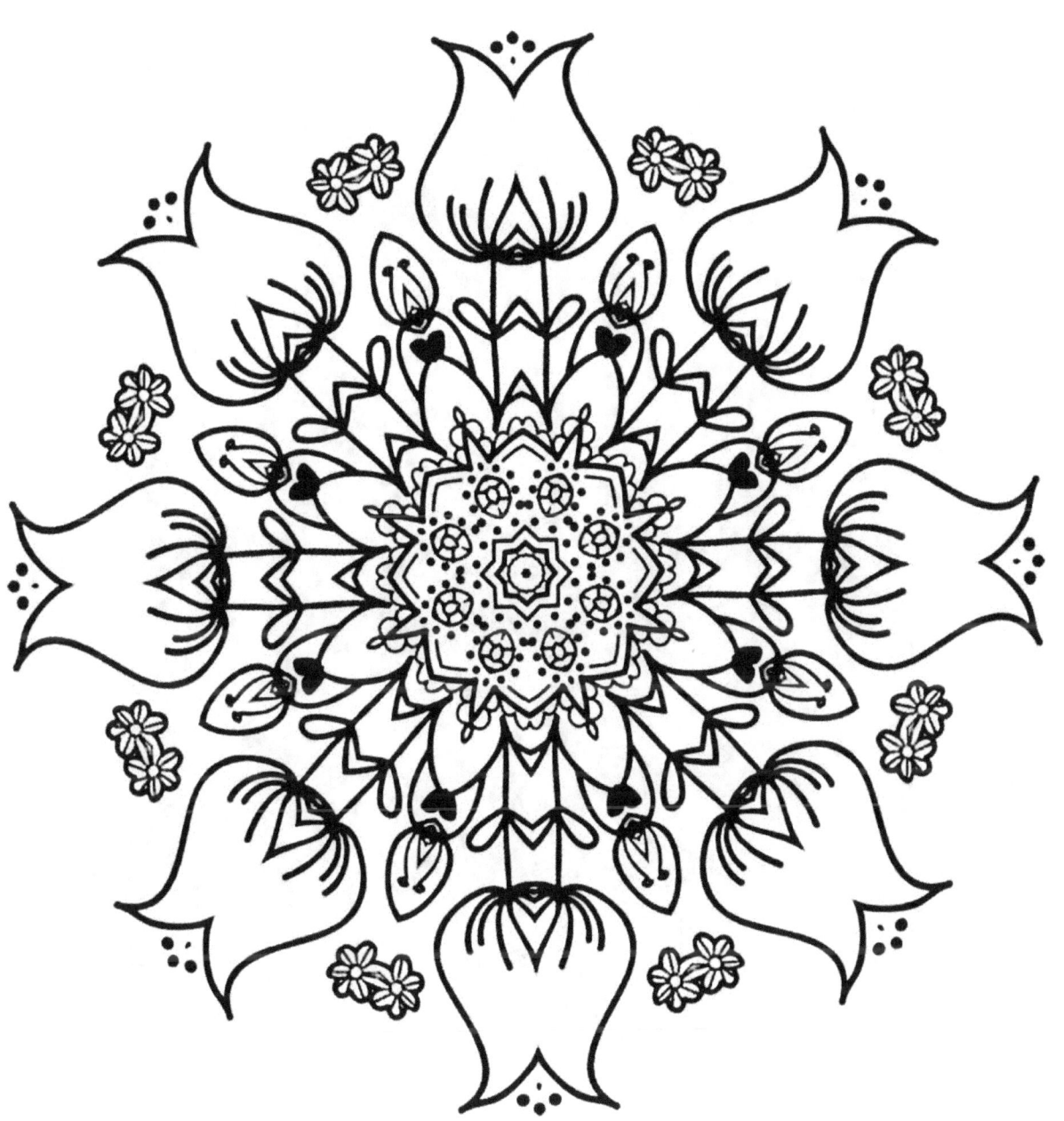

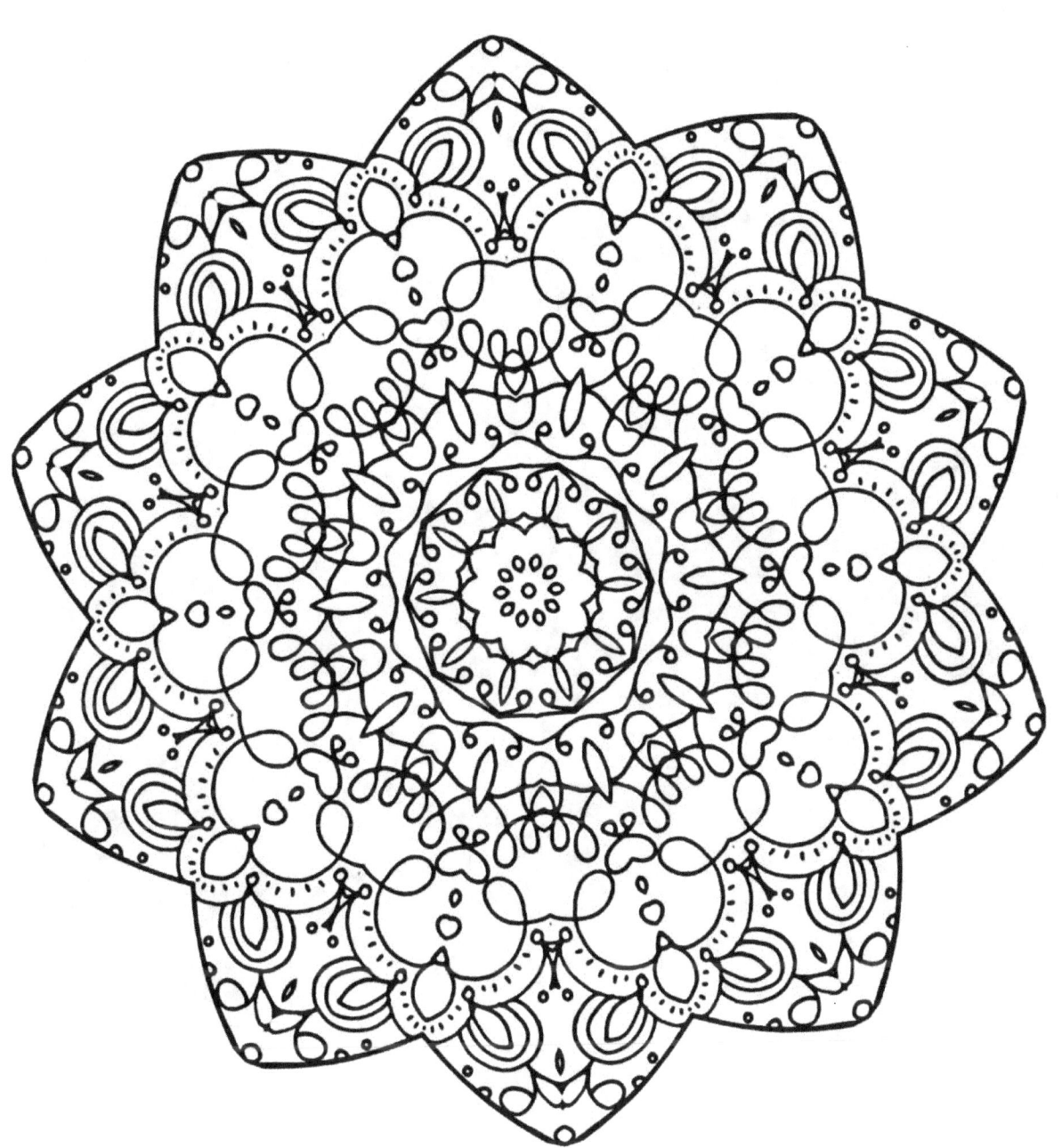

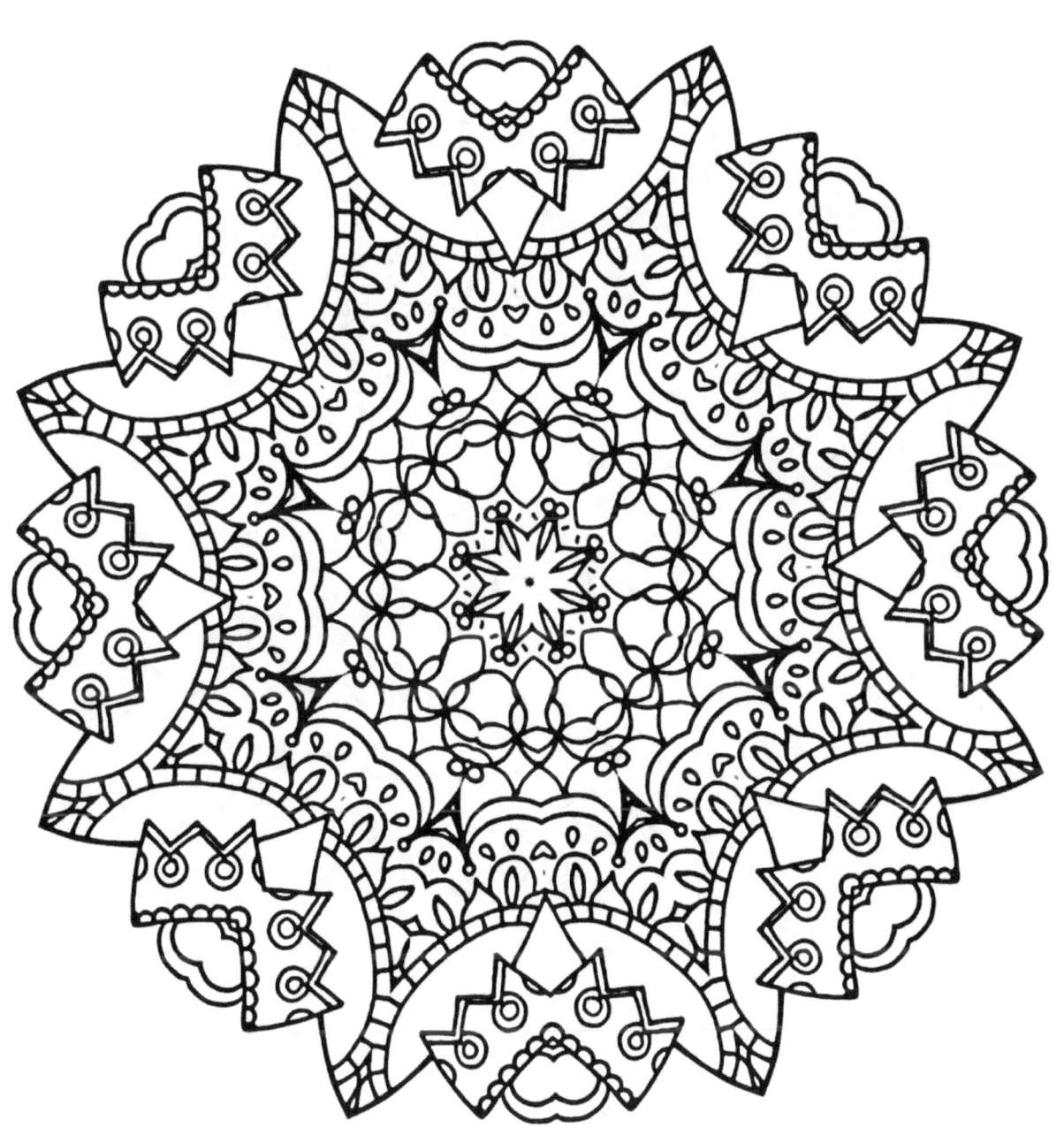

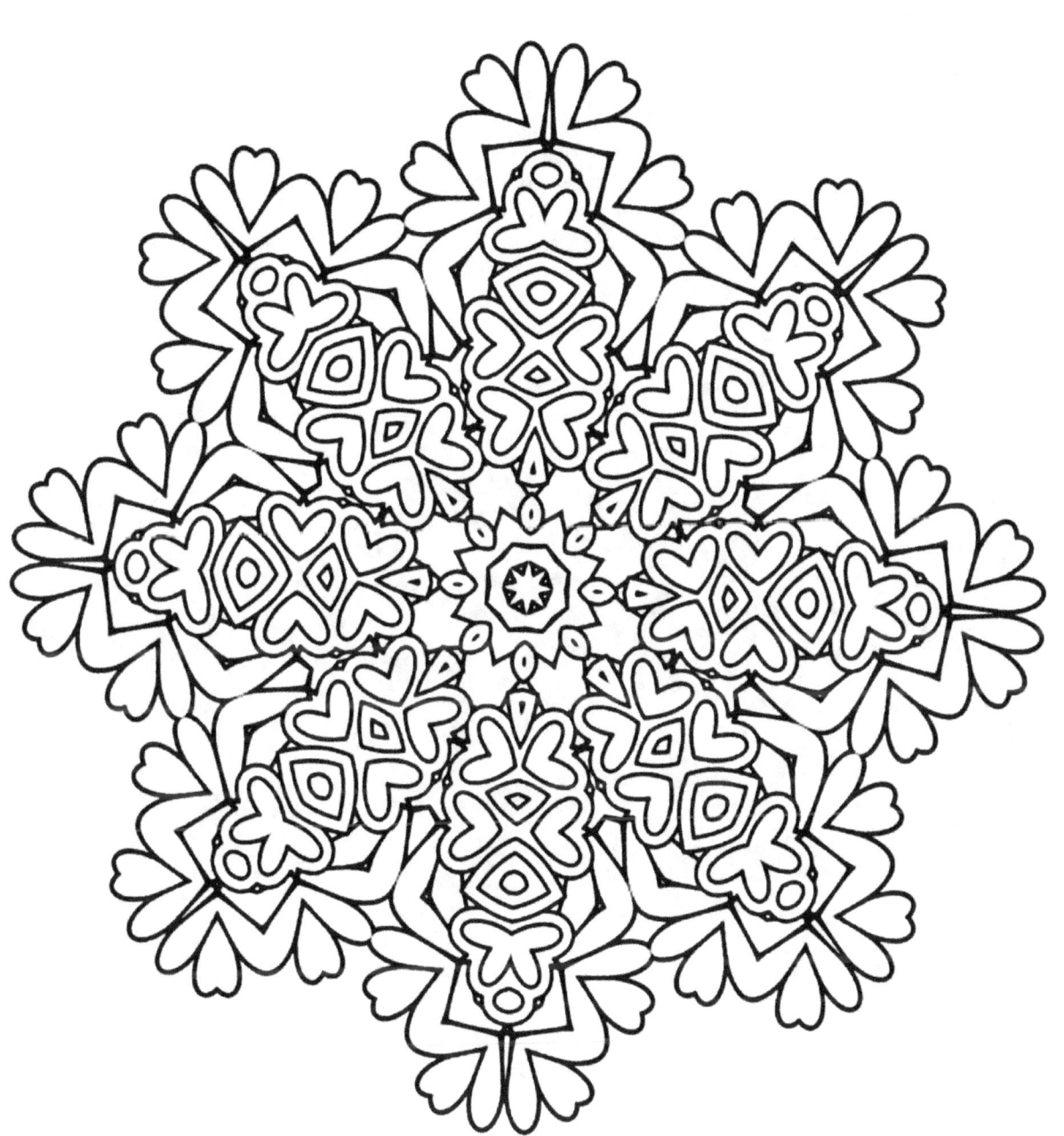

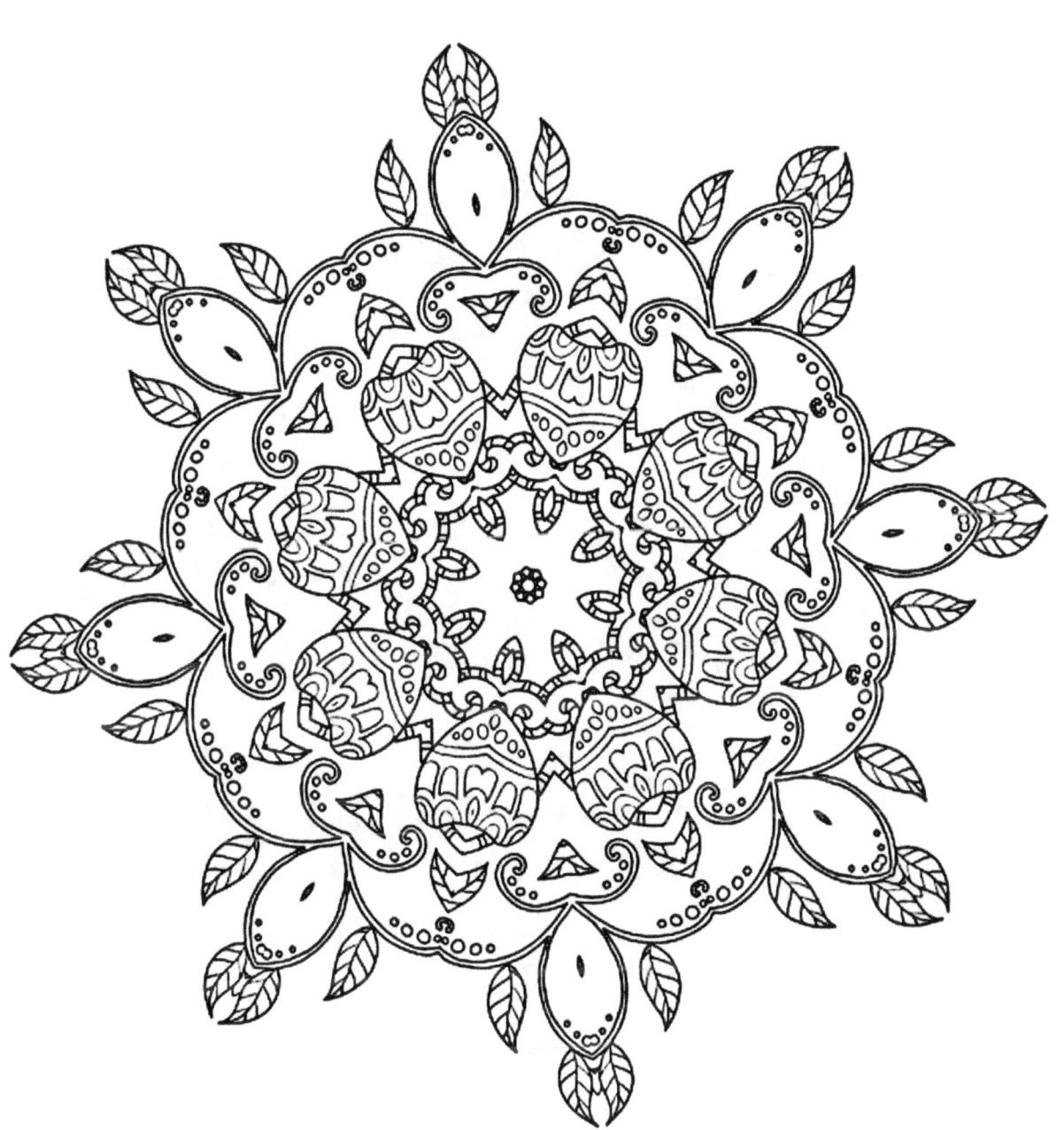

Thank you

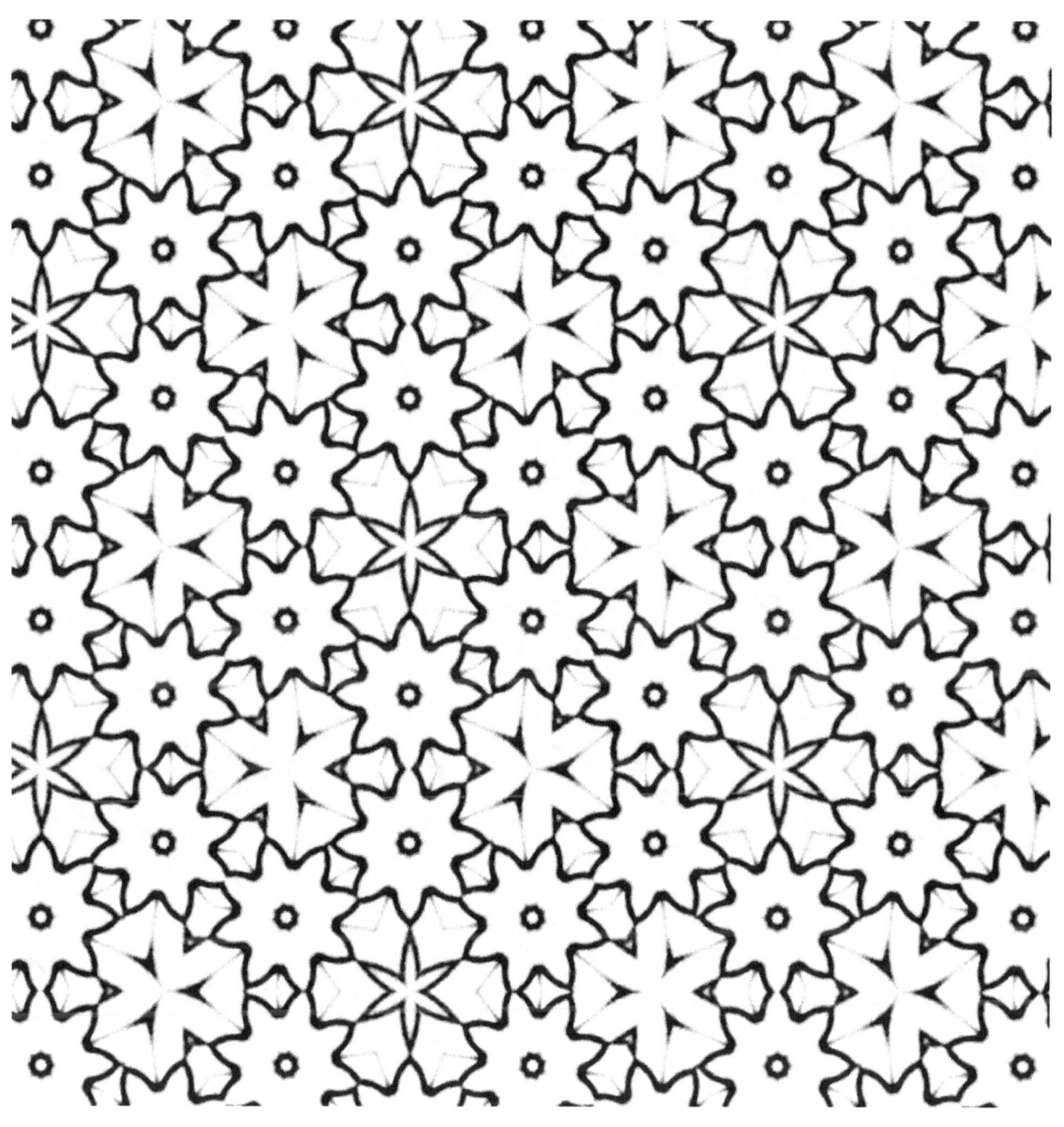

www.ingramcontent.com/pod-product-compliance
Lightning Source LLC
Chambersburg PA
CBHW081731170526
45167CB00009B/3786